Mesothelioma

Edited by Sonia Maciá

Published in London, United Kingdom

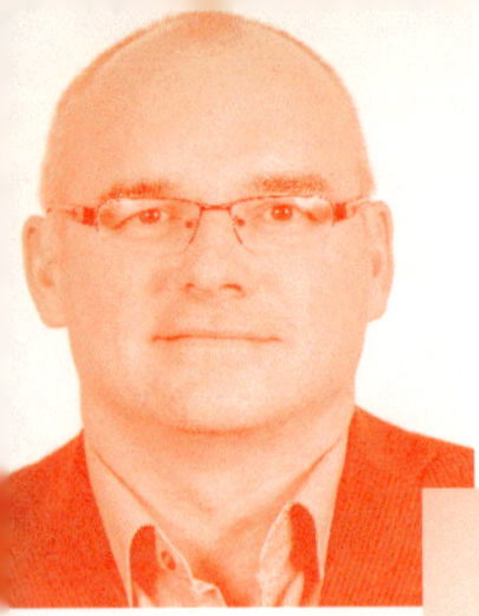
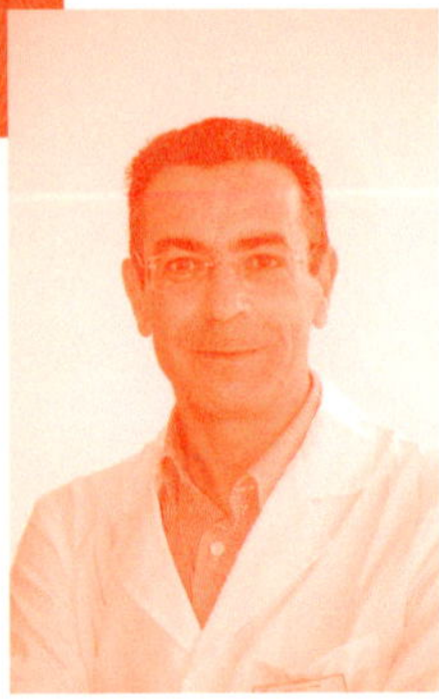
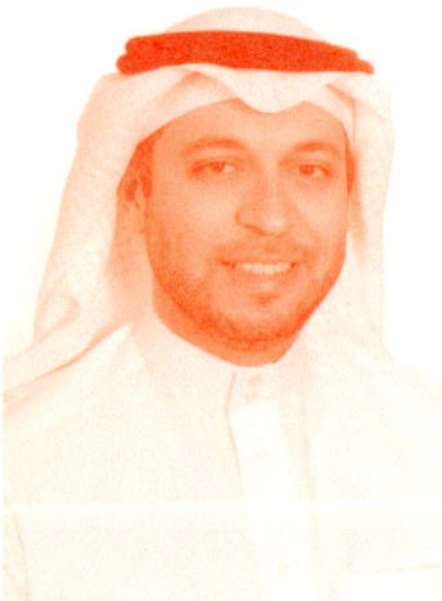
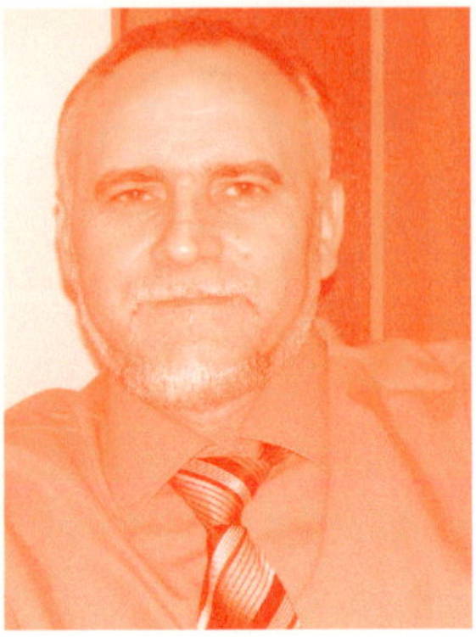
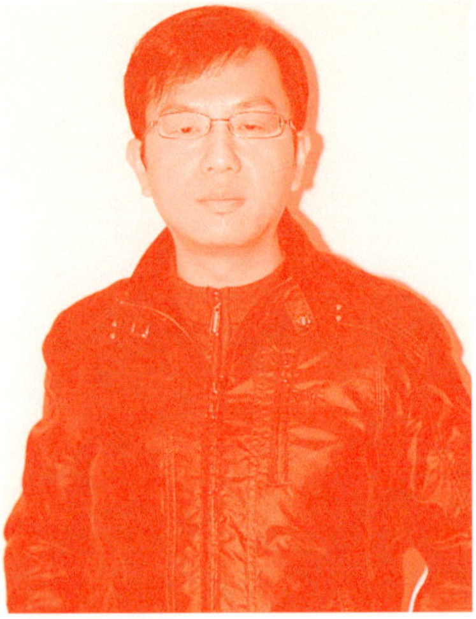
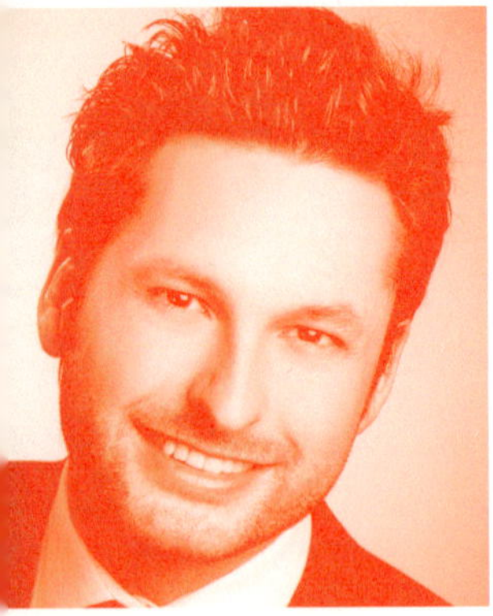
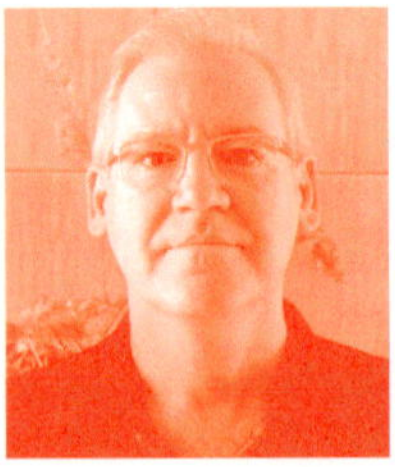

IntechOpen

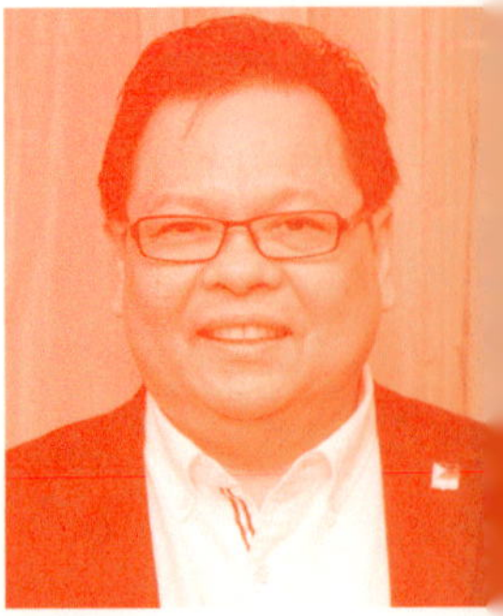
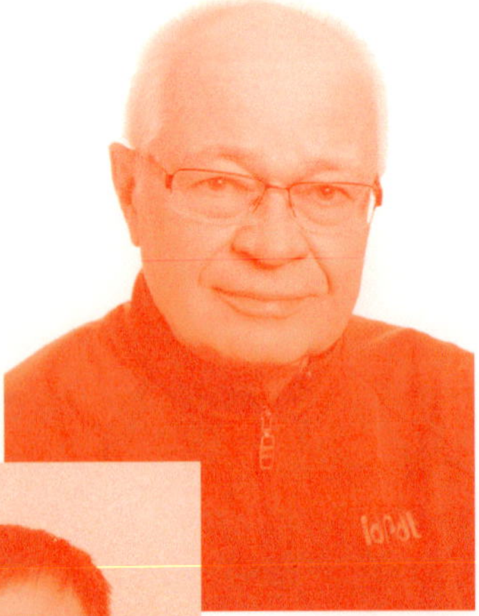
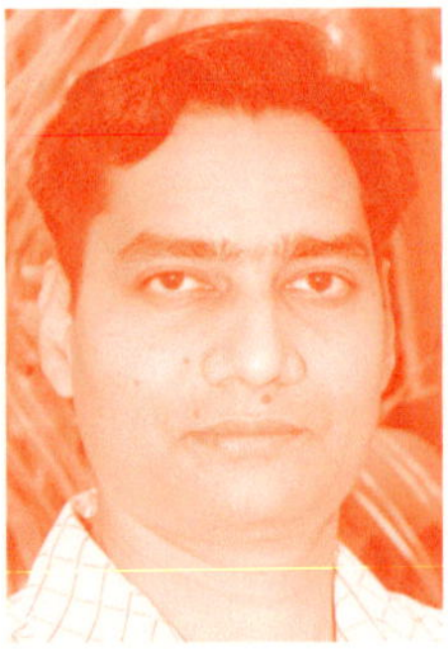
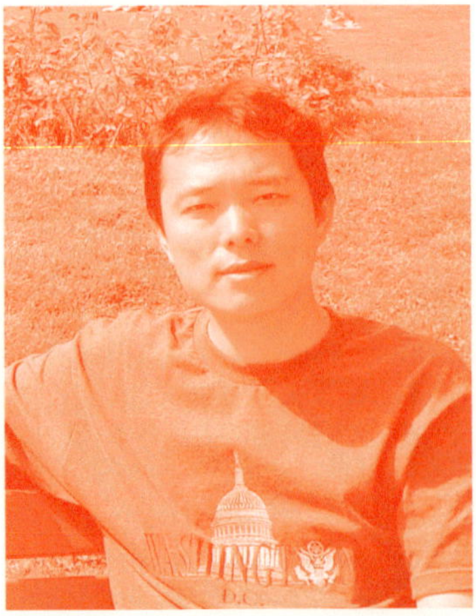
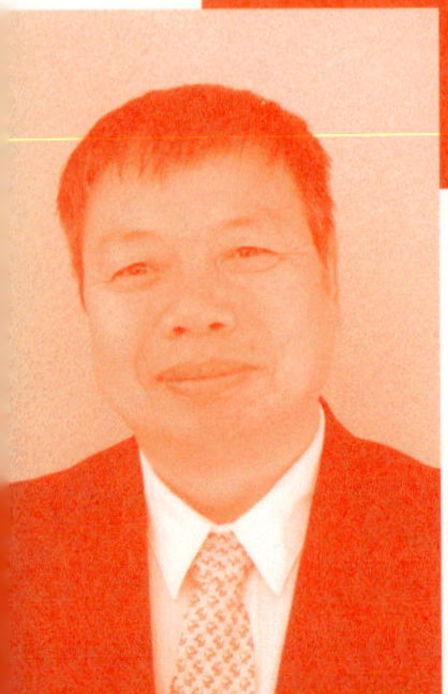
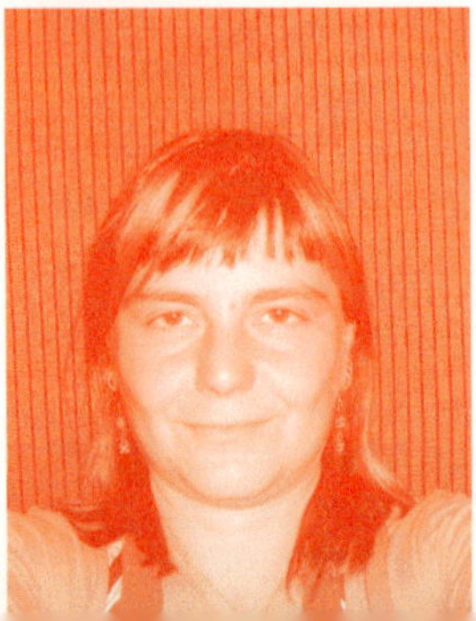

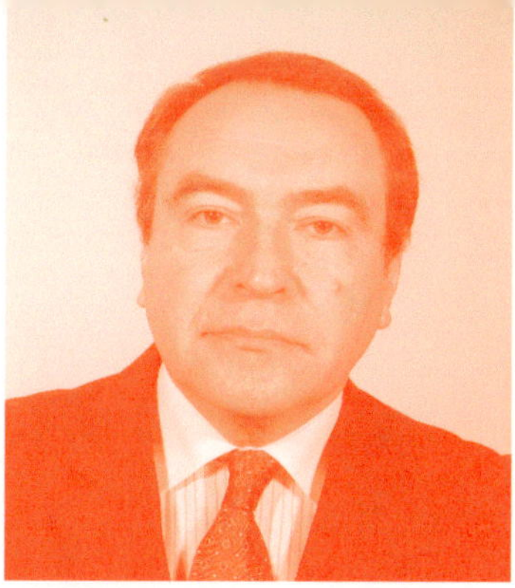
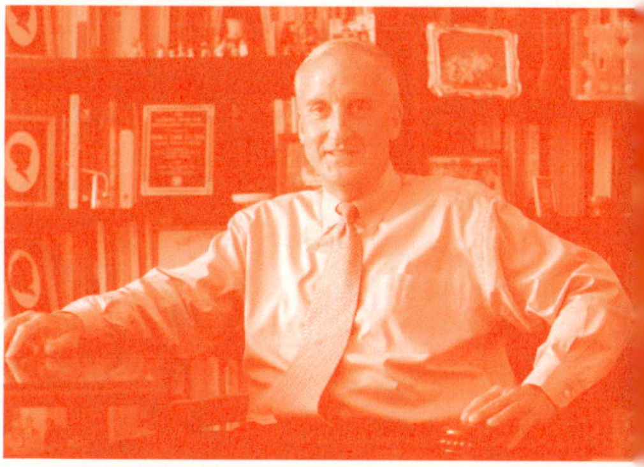
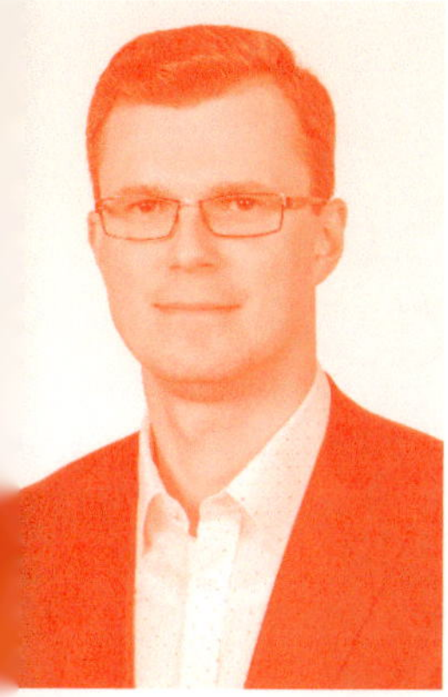
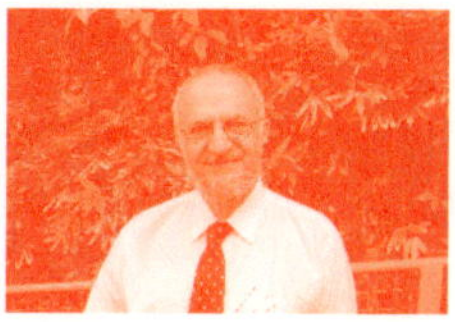
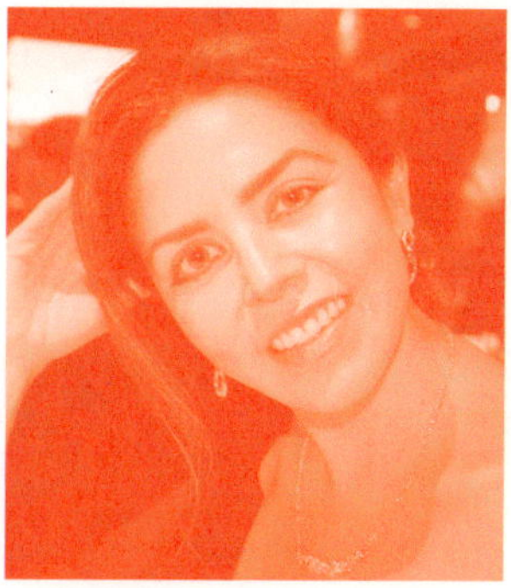

Supporting open minds since 2005

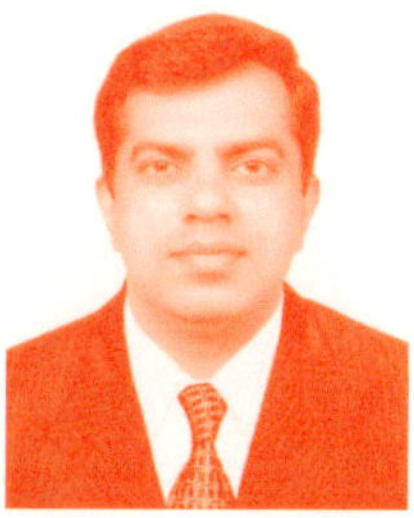
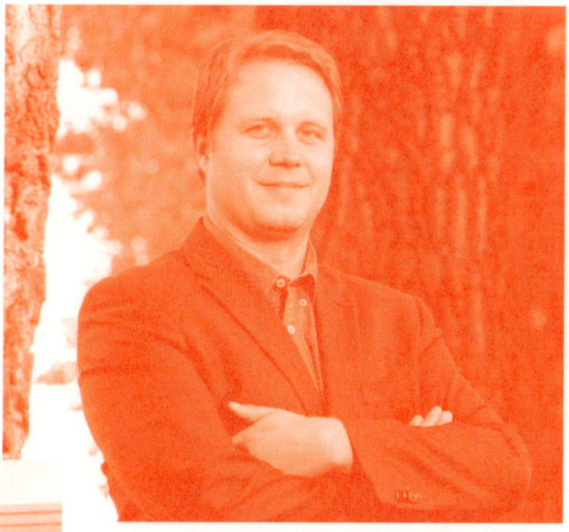
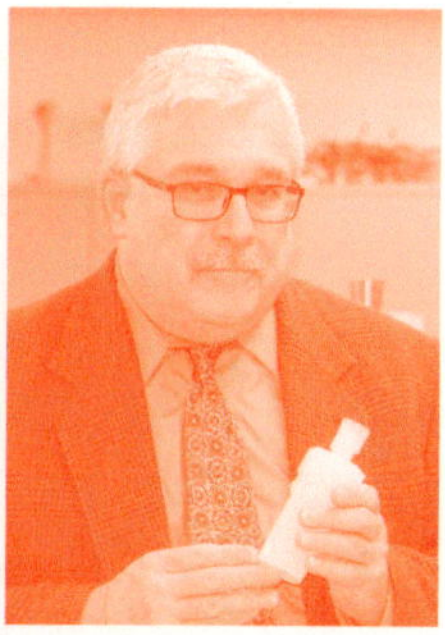
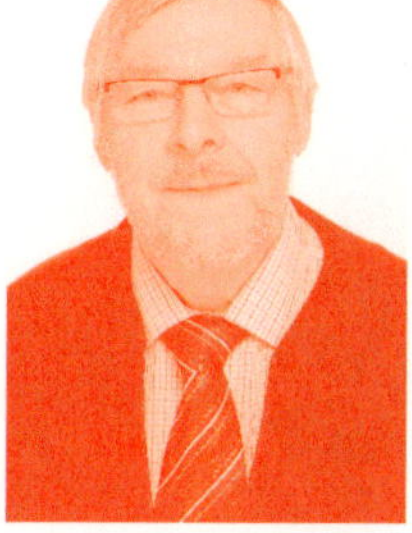
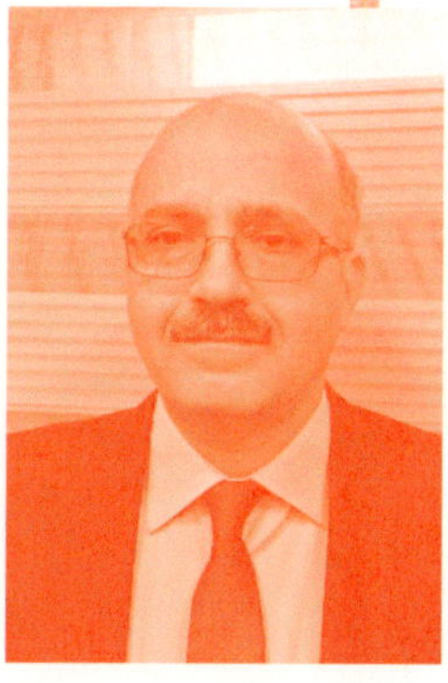
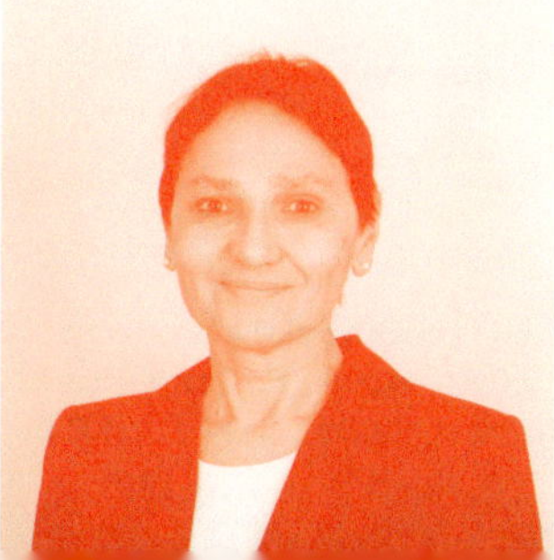
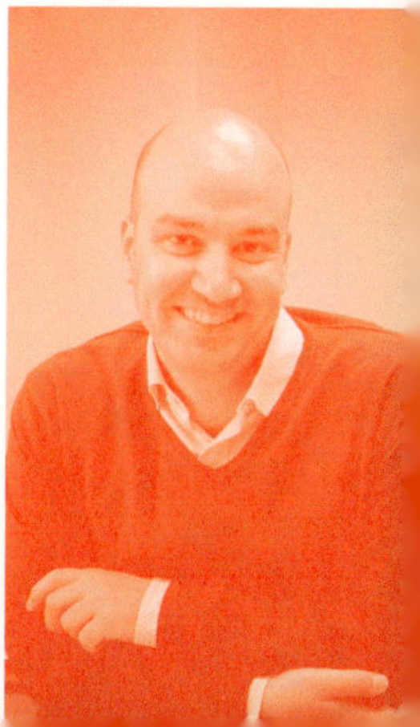

Mesothelioma
http://dx.doi.org/10.5772/intechopen.89396
Edited by Sonia Maciá

Contributors
Cristian Mesina, Mihaela-Iustina Mesina-Botoran, Theodor Viorel Dumitrescu, Mihai Calin Ciorbagiu, Cosmin Vasile Obleaga, Viji Shridhar, Jeremy Chien, Julian Molina, Derek B. Oien, Jeronimo Rodríguez-Cid, Rodrigo Rafael Flores-Mariñelarena, Assunta De Rienzo, Raphael Bueno, Benjamin Wadowski, David T. Severson, Muaiad Kittaneh, Jordyn Feinstein, Sonia Maciá, Vita Dolžan, Danijela Štrbac, Katja Goričar, Viljem Kovač

First published in London, United Kingdom, 2020 by IntechOpen
IntechOpen is the global imprint of INTECHOPEN LIMITED, registered in England and Wales, registration number: 11086078, 5 Princes Gate Court, London, SW7 2QJ, United Kingdom
Printed in Croatia

British Library Cataloguing-in-Publication Data
A catalogue record for this book is available from the British Library

Additional hard and PDF copies can be obtained from orders@intechopen.com

Mesothelioma
Edited by Sonia Maciá
p. cm.
Print ISBN 978-1-83968-154-7
Online ISBN 978-1-83968-155-4
eBook (PDF) ISBN 978-1-83968-156-1

For EU product safety concerns:
IN TECH d.o.o., Prolaz Marije Krucifikse Kozulić 3, 51000 Rijeka, Croatia, info@intechopen.com or visit our website at intechopen.com.

Meet the editor

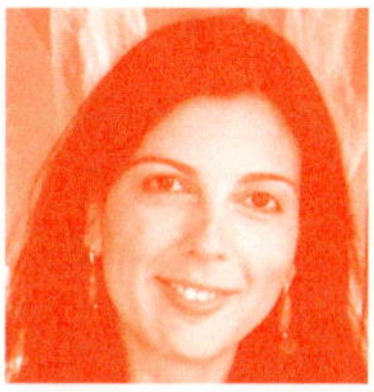

Sonia Maciá, MD, is an ESMO-certified Medical Oncologist. She obtained a master's degree in Pharmacoeconomy in 2018 from Universitat Pompeu Fabra Barcelona and a PhD in Lung Cancer from the Department of Clinical Medicine, University Miguel Hernández. Dr. Maciá worked as a practicing Medical Oncologist for nine years and then decided to devote her career to clinical research. In 2012 she joined Pivotal SL, a European CRO, as Medical Manager, being thereafter promoted to Medical Director. After a few months in a similar role at ICON Plc, she joined Highlight Therapeutics to work on clinical development, providing medical support to clinical trials in solid tumors. Dr. Maciá has submitted more than forty abstracts to international congresses, published more than thirty papers in peer-reviewed journals, and authored six book chapters.

Contents

Preface

Mesothelioma is a rare type of cancer belonging to those types of tumors for which there has been a lack of treatment advances in recent years. Overall, it is considered an extended disease with very limited aggressive treatment approaches.

This book presents a description of the most relevant topics on diagnosis, biomarkers, and treatment updates, including interesting discussion on prognostic features and novel therapies that are either approved or under clinical development.

Chapters provide insight into the current challenges in assessing predictive biomarkers and targeted therapies.

I thank the chapter authors for their valuable contributions and commitment to provide a clear and succinct overview of these topics.

Sonia Maciá
Medical Director,
Highlight Therapeutics,
Spain

Section 1

Introduction

Chapter 1

Mesothelioma, a Review of Current Guidelines

Sonia Maciá

Abstract

Mesothelioma is considered as a rare tumor originating in the mesothelial surfaces of pleura or, more rarely, in other sites such as peritoneum, which harbors a very poor prognosis. Despite clinical research efforts, lack of available therapies remains clear. Standard of care treatments and guidelines have not been evolved much along recent years. In this chapter, main guidelines will be reviewed, besides a systematic Pubmed review, with a focus on epidemiology, diagnosis tests, and approved local and systemic treatments, including most important advances. Searched terms included "mesothelioma," "ESMO and NCCN guidelines," "diagnosis," "surgery," "targeted therapy," "clinical trials," "palliative treatment," and "meta-analysis." First-line regimen recommendations have not evolved since the phase III pivotal study of cisplatin-pemetrexed was published, and this combination became the standard of care. Targeted therapies have brought disappointing results. However, recent clinical trial data with immunotherapies are bringing some light and may become a new paradigm in the following years.

Keywords: malignant mesothelioma, chemotherapy, pemetrexed, immunotherapy, clinical trials, nivolumab, pembrolizumab, targeted therapy

1. Introduction

Malignant mesothelioma (MM) is a fatal disease which originates in the mesothelial surfaces of pleura or, more rarely, in other sites such as peritoneum. Most cases have been classically linked to asbestos exposure; however, ionizing radiation may also increase the risk of mesothelioma [1].

Its prognosis is very poor and it is difficult to treat, mainly because most patients are diagnosed with advanced disease [1–3]. Despite clinical research efforts, lack of available therapies remains clear and median overall survival is still approximately 1 year, with only 10% patients alive 5 years after diagnosis. Standard of care treatments and guidelines have not been evolved much along recent years. In this chapter, NCCN and ESMO guidelines have been reviewed, besides an electronic search of the Pubmed database, with a focus on the phase II and III clinical trials, guidelines, meta-analysis, and systematic reviews regarding epidemiology, diagnosis tests, surgical approach, and approved local and systemic treatments, including most important advances. Searched terms included "mesothelioma," "ESMO and NCCN guidelines," "diagnosis," "surgery," "targeted therapy," "clinical trials," "palliative treatment," and "meta-analysis." First-line regimen recommendations have not evolved since the phase III pivotal study of cisplatin-pemetrexed was published, and this combination became the standard of care despite its modest benefit in survival. Pemetrexed seems to be the most active drug, but its use in the first-line setting limits its administration in further lines. However, a rechallenge may be done in responder patients, who might still get benefit [4].

Only few drugs have demonstrated a mild activity in refractory MM, and targeted therapies have provided disappointing results so far. However, recent clinical trial data with immunotherapies are bringing some light and may become a new paradigm in the following years.

2. Epidemiology

Malignant mesothelioma (MM) is a rare tumor, with an incidence of less than 5 out of 100,000 inhabitants in Europe [1]. Diagnosis is usually done when disease is well advanced, and patients have a high symptom burden [3]. Incidence has decreased along the last decades globally worldwide. Mesothelioma has been typically related to asbestos exposure, which is the most well-known risk factor, although the latency period can be long, with a latency period being approximately 40 years, although in some cases, it may be as long as 60–70 years. Recent reports have suggested that also ionizing radiation may have a role, such as in patients previously treated with radiotherapy (RT). Other studies also suggest that erionite (which may be found in travel roads) increases the risk of MM. Smoking is not a risk factor. There may be a genetic risk in patients with BRCA-1 mutation [5–7].

The most common type of mesothelioma is malignant pleural mesothelioma, being up to 70% cases, followed by peritoneal (30%) and pericardial mesothelioma (1–2%) [2]. According to histology, there are three subtypes: epithelial, sarcomatoid, and biphasic [3], with epithelial subtype having a better prognosis.

Prevalence is highly linked to mortality, and mesothelioma is an unmet medical need due to its very poor prognosis, having a median overall survival of approximately 9–12 months, with only very modest improvements in survival over time [8].

3. Diagnosis

Most common symptoms include dyspnea, thoracic pain, and weight loss. Usually unilateral effusions are observed. A detailed occupational history is key, checking asbestos exposure among other previously exposed potential risk factors. Patients often present with advanced disease, but without distant metastases, as local implants or effusion cause pain and/or dyspnea. Brain metastases are rare [3].

Diagnosis assessments include chest X-ray, computed tomography (CT) scan of chest and upper abdomen, and thoracentesis, with examination of the pleural effusion and general laboratory blood tests [1]. Citology samples from pleural effusion are frequently negative or inconclusive, hence, histology may bring some further light for a more accurate diagnosis. Some biomarkers may be helpful, including calretinin, WT-1, D2-40, and citokeratyn 5/6, being negative in mesothelioma and positive in lung adenocarcinoma [9]. In order to obtain adequate histology, a thoracoscopy is highly recommended to optimally stage and to allow pleural fluid evacuation (with or without pleurodesis) [9, 10]. Mesothelioma can be difficult to identify and distinguish from benign pleural lesions and from other malignancies; it is therefore recommended to obtain biopsies from the tissue of both abnormal and normal appearance. When a thoracoscopy is not feasible or contraindicated, ultrasound-guided true-cut biopsies are a good alternative [10].

4. Pathology

MM comprises a heterogeneous group of tumors, which are mainly classified as three subtypes (epithelioid, biphasic, and sarcomatoid), despite the numerous variants that are described in the 2004 WHO classification [9].

Diagnosis samples may be obtained from pleural effusions, pleural biopsies, and surgical samples [1, 8–10]. Cytological diagnosis from effusion samples may be feasible, but sensitivity is highly variant, with variable atypia (usually low grade). Therefore, usually tissue biopsies with immunohistochemistry analysis are pivotal for confirmatory diagnosis.

Standardly used and most recommended biomarkers for diagnosis include calretinin, cytokeratin 5/6, WT1, and podoplanin (D240). For non-small cell adcenocarcinoma, the most useful markers are TTF1, CEA, and EP4 [8].

5. Staging

Staging procedures are aimed to describe anatomical extent correlating with prognostic features, which is key in order to make treatment decisions. Standard procedures for staging include chest and abdomen CT with contrast and PET/CT (for those patients who may undergo surgery). Video-assisted thoracoscopy (VATS) is recommended if contralateral disease is suspected [3].

Patients should be evaluated by a multidisciplinary committee, including oncologist, radiation oncologist, pathologist, pulmonologist, diagnostic imaging specialist, and surgeon.

The limitation of most classifications is their inaccuracy in describing tumor (T-) and node (N-) extent. The most recent staging system was presented by the International Mesothelioma Interest Group (IMIG) [11]. However, it failed to be an independent prognostic factor when analyzed in the clinical setting using multivariate analysis [11–14]. Hence, further workup is needed in order to get an accurate and prognostic staging system.

If a surgical resection is planned, either mediastinoscopy or endobronchial ultrasound of mediastinal lymph nodes are recommended [15]. Besides, two additional tests may be useful if suggested by imaging: laparoscopy in order to rule out any transdiaphragmatic extension and chest MRI to check vascular involvement [14–17].

6. Treatment for mesothelioma

6.1 First-line therapy for mesothelioma

Chemotherapy is recommended as the sole therapy for patients with ECOG 0–2 who are not amenable for surgery. For patients with ECOG 3–4, best supportive care is strongly recommended.

Chemotherapy has a role in the palliative treatment of advanced mesothelioma, getting an improvement of symptoms and modest benefit in survival. Standard first-line treatment is based on platinum doublets, with either pemetrexed or raltitrexed [18, 19], being cisplatin/pemetrexed the only FDA-approved regimen. This combination was investigated in a phase III trial comparing cisplatin/pemetrexed vs. cisplatin monotherapy, getting a benefit in survival by 2.8 months (12.1 vs. 9.3 months, $P = 0.02$) [18].

Carboplatin may be used as an alternative to cisplatin, particularly in fragile patients, with no significant differences in survival and a better safety profile [20, 21].

Clinical research has been trying to look for an improvement with the addition of several agents; however, several phase II trials have failed to demonstrate improvement over standard treatment with the addition of antioangiogenics such as bevacizumab or sunitinib [22, 23]. However, a phase III trial compared cisplatin/pemetrexed with or without bevacizumab in patients who were suitable for receiving bevacizumab (ECOG 0–2 with no history of bleeding or thrombosis). Experimental arm was better in terms of survival, with a benefit by 2.7 months (18.8 vs. 16.1 months, P = 0.0167). Grade 3–4 adverse events were more common in the experimental arm, 71 vs. 62%, with more cases of hypertension, grade 3 proteinuria and grade 3–4 thromboembolic events in the bevacizumab arm. The NCCN guidelines then recommends cisplatin/pemetrexed plus bevacizumab followed by maintenance bevacizumab in patients without contraindications [24].

6.2 Second-line therapy for mesothelioma

There is a lack of treatment options in the second line and beyond setting, this being an important medical need with no standard of care yet. Pemetrexed as single agent when compared with the best supportive care was not able to provide an improvement in survival [25]. Vinorelbine showed a benefit in terms of responses in several small phase II trials [26].

Both immunotherapies and targeted therapies are under evaluation as well, but they have not been yielded into approval [27, 28]. In the absence of the standard second-line or further-line therapy, it is recommended that patients are enrolled into clinical trials. Recent data suggest that checkpoint inhibitors may have a role in this setting, with a response rate slightly higher than that previously obtained by other agents [3].

Checkpoint inhibitors target the programmed death-1 (PD-1) receptor, which improves tumor immunity. Both nivolumab and pembrolizumab target PD-1 receptors, but testing this receptor is not required [29].

6.3 Immunotherapy and targeted therapies

Some immunotherapies have been tested or are under clinical development for MPM, including antibodies blocking immune checkpoints that function as negative regulators of T-cell function, cytotoxic T-lymphocyte-associated antigen 4 (CTLA4), programmed death 1 (PD-1), and programmed death ligand 1 (PD-L1). However, there is still a lack of strong support for their use.

In two nonrandomized studies, the anti-CTLA4 antibody tremelimumab showed preliminary evidence of activity in patients with previously treated mesothelioma [28, 30]. Thereafter, a randomized, placebo-controlled study investigated tremelimumab in patients with mesothelioma (the DETERMINE trial). This trial did not meet the primary end point of OS, as we did not find statistically significant differences in OS between the tremelimumab group [median OS 7.7 months (95% CI: 6.8–8.9)] and the placebo group [median OS 7.3 months (95% CI: 5.9–8.7)] [31].

In the KEYNOTE-028 trial, previously treated patients with PD-L1-positive MPM received pembrolizumab 10 mg/kg every 2 weeks for up to 2 years or until confirmed progression or unacceptable toxicity. Five of 25 patients (20%) had a partial response (objective response rate of 20%) and 13 (52%) patients had stable disease. Additionally, there was a maintained clinical benefit, with a median duration of response 12.0 months (95% CI: 3.7 not reached) [32, 33]. The NivoMes study, which evaluated nivolumab in unselected patients with previously treated mesothelioma reported response rates of 28%. The JAVELIN study of the anti-PDL-1 antibody avelumab in unselected patients with previously treated mesothelioma reported a response rate of 9.4% with a median PFS of 17.1 weeks. Subgroup analysis in the PD-L1-positive population (cutoff > 5%) showed a response rate of 14% [34]. Novel vaccine approaches using MPM neoantigens identified by gene sequencing are also entering clinical trial on the basis of early animal studies [33].

As a summary, preliminary data on PD-1- and PD-L1-targeting monoclonal antibodies in MPM suggest that immunotherapy with single agents may have some benefit, possibly because of its complex biology.

6.4 Radiotherapy

Administering RT to the entire pleural surface without damaging radiosensitive sites and keeping a good safety profile is very challenging. Radiotherapy (RT) is used in different settings as treatment for MM: palliative, adjuvant, and as part of a multimodality treatment.

As palliative treatment for pain relief bronchial obstruction or other disease related symptoms, there is no strong evidence to support its use; however, it may be recommended in cases of infiltration of the chest wall, administered in short courses such as 1 × 10 or 3 × 8 Gy [35], always understanding that dose of radiation should be based on its purpose.

6.4.1 Pre- and postoperative RT

Limited evidence is available, extracted from retrospective studies only. In general results are poor, in terms of disease control rate, because of the complex growth patterns of the disease. Furthermore, its safety profile is poor due to the wide field size and neighboring vital organs. The introduction of intensity-modulated RT (IMRT) seem to overcome most of these issues and allow the remaining tumor tissue to be properly irradiated. Preliminary results adjuvant IMRT seemed particularly promising. Further studies are needed to better establish the role of RT. Recent studies have underlined the importance of RT technique, both in terms of local control and toxicity. It is therefore recommended that RT is delivered in specialized centers (expert advice) [36, 37].

6.5 Surgery

Surgery may be recommended for patients with stage I to IIIA disease who are in good conditions and are medically operable. A careful assessment before proceeding to surgery is strongly recommended [1, 3].

Objectives of surgery are staging, palliative, and, more uncommonly, curative intent.

6.5.1 Surgery with radical intent

It cannot be considered to have a real radical intention, as its objective is actually obtaining a macroscopic resection removing as much tumor as possible since it is virtually impossible to obtain free resection margins [1]. It can include pleurectomy/decortication (complete removal of involved pleural and all gross tumor) or extrapleural pneumonectomy, including in bloc resection of pleura, lung diaphragm, and often also part of pericardium [38].

Some studies assessed a second-step surgery, following an induction chemotherapy, which is reported as a trimodality approach. Different combined modality regimens have been investigated.

The European Organization for Research and Treatment of Cancer (EORTC) analyzed trimodality therapy in a phase II trial (EORTC 08031). Patients with MM (up to stage cT3N1M0) received induction chemotherapy (cisplatin and pemetrexed × 3) followed by surgery within 21–56 days. Forty-two out of 57 (73.7%) included patients could undergo surgery. Survival figures were positive, with an overall survival of 18.4 months and 13.9 months progression-free survival. Operative mortality was 6.4% [39].

Other phase II trial with a similar design was performed in the USA and included 77 patients, achieving an overall survival of 16.8 months, with an operative mortality of 7% [40].

Although trimodal therapy seemed feasible in selected patients with promising results, it was further evaluated in a phase III trial in the UK with negative results (MARS1 study). In this trial, mortality was as high as 18.8%, with only 45% patients undergoing surgery after induction treatment, and with a lower survival for patients undergoing surgery compared to the control arm where patients received only the induction therapy (14 vs. 19 months) [41].

However, a systematic review performed afterward, including 34 studies from 26 institutions, found highly variant results, with the median survival ranging from 9.4 to 27.5 months and surgical morbidity from 22 to 82%. Probably, it may be explained by different surgical approaches, variability in terms of surgeon's prior experience, and heterogeneity of included patients, but some patients may get benefit from this treatment [42]. A multidisciplinary team with sufficient experience should provide recommendations on the suitability of patients for trimodality therapy.

6.5.2 Surgery for staging and palliation

Control pleural effusion, talc poudrage, or even decortication in a captured lung may be performed through surgery. One study compared VATS (partial) pleurectomy vs. standard talc poudrage in 196 patients. There was no benefit in terms of survival, but control of pleural effusion and quality of life were significantly better for experimental arm at 6 and 12 months [43].

7. Conclusions

This chapter shows a review of both NCCN and ESMO guidelines besides PubMed available literature. Mesothelioma is one of those tumors with less advanced in the recent years, probably due to its aggressive nature and the limited incidence, which makes clinical research more time consuming. This is considered still as a medical need due to the lack of treatment options beyond the second line. However, research is improving and some immunooncology agents have started to show a small but significant benefit in terms of survival.

Conflict of interest

The author declares no conflict of interest.

DOI: http://dx.doi.org/10.5772/intechopen.93569

Author details

Sonia Maciá
Highlight Therapeutics, Spain

*Address all correspondence to: smacia@yahoo.com;
smacia@highlighttherapeutics.com

References

[1] Baas P, Fennell D, Kerr KM, Van Schil PE, Haas RL, Peters S. Malignant pleural mesothelioma: ESMO clinical practice guidelines. Annals of Oncology. 2015;**26**(Suppl 5):v31-v39

[2] Alpert N, van Gerwen M, Taioli E. Epidemiology of mesothelioma in the 21st century in Europe and the United States, 40 years after restricted/banned asbestos use. Transl Lung Cancer Res. 2020 Feb;**9**(Suppl 1):S28-S38

[3] Ettinger D, Wood D. On behalf of nccn malignant pleural mesothelioma. NCCN Clinical Practice Guidelines in Oncology. 2019 November 27. https://www.nccn.org/professionals/physician_gls/pdf/mpm.pdf

[4] Di Noia V, Vita E, Ferrara M, et al. Malignant pleural mesothelioma: Is tailoring the second-line therapy really "raising the Bar?". Current Treatment Options in Oncology. 2019;**20**(3):23. Published 2019 February 21. DOI: 10.1007/s11864-019-0616-7

[5] Xu R, Barg FK, Emmet EA, et al. Association between mesothelioma and non-occupational asbestos exposure: Systematic review and meta-analysis. Environmental Health. 2018;**17**:90

[6] Carbone M, Kanodia S, Chao A, et al. Consensus report of the 2015 Weinman international conference on mesothelioma. Journal of Thoracic Oncology. 2016;**11**:1246-1262

[7] Betti M, Casalone E, Ferrante D, et al. Germline mutations in DNA repair genes predispose asbestos-exposed patients to malignant pleural mesothelioma. Cancer Letters. 2017;**405**:38-45

[8] Yang H, Testa JR, Carbone M. Mesothelioma epidemiology, carcinogenesis and pathogenesis. Current Treatment Options in Oncology. 2008;**9**:147-157. DOI: 10.1007/s11864-008-0067-z

[9] Paintal A, Raparia K, Zakowski MF, Nayar R. The diagnosis of malignant mesothelioma in effusion citology: A reappraisal and results of a multi-institution survey. Cancer Cytopathology. 2013;**121**:703-707

[10] Maskell NA, Gleeson FV, Davies RJ. Standard pleural biopsy versus CT-guided cutting-needle biopsy for diagnosis of malignant disease in pleural effusions: A randomised controlled trial. Lancet. 2003;**361**:1326-1330

[11] Greillier L, Cavailles A, Fraticelli A, et al. Accuracy of pleural biopsy using thoracoscopy for the diagnosis of histologic subtype in patients with malignant pleural mesothelioma. Cancer. 2007;**110**:2248-2252

[12] Churg A, Roggli VL, Galateau-Salle F, et al. Tumours of the pleura: Mesothelial tumours. In: Travis WD, Brambilla E, Muller-Hermelink HK, Harris CC, editors. Pathology and Genetics of Tumours of the Lung, Pleura, Thymus and Heart. Lyon, France: IARC; 2004 (World Health Organization Classification of Tumours 10: 128-136)

[13] Husain AN, Colby T, Ordonez N, et al. Guidelines for pathologic diagnosis of malignant mesothelioma: 2012 update of the consensus statement from the International Mesothelioma Interest Group. Archives of Pathology & Laboratory Medicine. 2013;**137**:647-667

[14] Rusch VW. A proposed new international TNM staging system for malignant pleural mesothelioma. From the International Mesothelioma Interest Group. Chest. 1995;**108**:1122-1128

[15] Rice DC, Steliga MA, Stewart J, et al. Endoscopic ultrasound-guided fine needle aspiration for staging og malignant pleural mesothelioma. Ann Thorac Srug. 2009;**88**:862-868

[16] Nowak AK, Armato SG III, Ceresoli GL, et al. Imaging in pleural mesothelioma: A review of imaging research presented at the 9th International Meeting of the International Mesothelioma Interest Group. Lung Cancer. 2010;**70**:1-6

[17] Tammilehto L, Kivisaari L, Salminen US, et al. Evaluation of the clinical TNM staging system for malignant pleural mesothelioma: An assessment in 88 patients. Lung Cancer. 1995;**12**:25-34

[18] Vogelzang NJ, Rusthoven JJ, Symanowski J, et al. Phase III study of pemetrexed in combination with cisplatin versus cisplatin alone in patients with malignant pleural mesothelioma. Journal of Clinical Oncology. 2003;**21**:2636-2644

[19] van Meerbeeck JP, Gaafar R, Manegold C, et al. Randomized phase III study of cisplatin with or without raltitrexed in patients with malignant pleural mesothelioma: An intergroup study of the European Organisation for Research and Treatment of Cancer Lung Cancer Group and the National Cancer Institute of Canada. Journal of Clinical Oncology. 2005;**23**:6881-6889

[20] Santoro A, O'Brien ME, Stahel RA, et al. Pemetrexed plus cisplatin or pemetrexed plus carboplatin for chemonaive patients with malignant pleural mesothelioma: Results of the International Expanded Access Program. Journal of Thoracic Oncology. 2008;**3**:756-763

[21] Ceresoli GL, Castagneto B, Zucali PA, et al. Pemetrexed plus carboplatin in elderly patients with malignant pleural mesothelioma: Combined analysis of two phase II trials. British Journal of Cancer. 2008;**99**:51-56

[22] Kindler HL, Karrison TG, Gandara DR, et al. Multicenter, double-blind, placebo-controlled, randomized phase II trial of gemcitabine/cisplatin plus bevacizumab or placebo in patients with malignant mesothelioma. Journal of Clinical Oncology. 2012;**30**:2509-2515

[23] Nowak AK, Millward MJ, Creaney J, et al. A phase II trial of intermittent sunitinib maleate as second-line therapy in progressive malignant pleural mesothelioma. Journal of Thoracic Oncology. 2012;**7**:1449-1456

[24] Zalcman G, Mazieres J, Margery J, et al. Bevacizumab for newly diagnosed pleural mesothelioma in the mesothelioma Avastin Cisplatin Pemetrexed Study (MAPS): A randomized, controlled, open-label, phase 3 trial. Lancet. 2016;**387**:1405-1414

[25] Manegold C, Symanowski J, Gatzemeier U, et al. Second-line (post-study) chemotherapy received by patients treated in the phase III trial of pemetrexed plus cisplatin versus cisplatin alone in malignant pleural mesothelioma. Annals of Oncology. 2005;**16**:923-927

[26] Stebbing J, Powles T, McPherson K, et al. The efficacy and safety of weekly vinorelbine in relapsed malignant pleural mesothelioma. Lung Cancer. 2009;**63**:94-97

[27] Hassan R, Miller AC, Sharon E, et al. Major cancer regressions in mesothelioma after treatment with an anti-mesothelin immunotoxin and immune suppression. Science Translational Medicine. 2013;**5**:208ra147

[28] Calabro L, Morra A, Fonsatti E, et al. Tremelimumab for patients with chemotherapy-resistant advanced malignant mesothelioma: An

open-label, single-arm, phase 2 trial. The Lancet Oncology. 2013;**14**:1104-1111

[29] Hom L, Spigel DR, Vokes EE, et al. Nivolumab versus docetaxel in previously treated patients with advanced non small cell lung cancer: Two year outcomes from two randomized, open label, phase III trials (checkmate 017 and checkmate 057). Journal of Clinical Oncology. 2017;**35**:3924-3933

[30] Calabro L, Morra A, Fonsatti E, et al. Efficacy and safety of an intensified schedule of tremelimumab for chemotherapy-resistant malignant mesothelioma: An open-label, singlearm, phase 2 study. The Lancet Respiratory Medicine. 2015;**3**:301-309

[31] Maio M, Scherpereel A, Calabro L, et al. Tremelimumab as second-line or third-line treatment in relapsed malignant mesothelioma (DETERMINE): A multicentre, international, randomised, double-blind, placebo-controlled phase 2b trial. The Lancet Oncology. 2017;**18**:1261-1273

[32] Alley EW, Lopez J, Santoro A, et al. Clinical safety and activity of pembrolizumab in patients with malignant pleural mesothelioma (KEYNOTE-028): Preliminary results from a non-randomised, open-label, phase 1b trial. The Lancet Oncology. 2017;**18**:623-630

[33] Namikawa K, Yamazaki N. Targeted therapy and immunotherapy for melanoma in Japan. Current Treatment Options in Oncology. 2019;**20**(1):7. Published 2019 January 24. DOI: 10.1007/s11864-019-0607-8

[34] Quispel-Janssen J, Zago G, Schouten R, et al. OA13.01 a phase II study of nivolumab in malignant pleural mesothelioma (NivoMes): With translational research (TR) biopies. Journal of Thoracic Oncology. 2017;**12**:S292-S293

[35] MacLeod N, Chalmers A, O'Rourke N, et al. Is radiotherapy useful for treating pain in mesothelioma? A phase II trial. Journal of Thoracic Oncology. 2015;**10**:944-950

[36] Rusch VW, Rosenzweig K, Venkatraman E, et al. A phase II trial of surgical resection and adjuvant high-dose hemithoracic radiation for malignant pleural mesothelioma. The Journal of Thoracic and Cardiovascular Surgery. 2001;**122**:788-795

[37] Allen AM, Czerminska M, Jänne PA, et al. Fatal pneumonitis associated with intensity-modulated radiation therapy for mesothelioma. International Journal of Radiation Oncology, Biology, Physics. 2006;**65**:640-645

[38] Rice D, Rusch V, Pass H, et al. Recommendations for uniform definitions of surgical techniques for malignant pleural mesothelioma: A consensus report of the international association for the study of lung cancer international staging committee and the international mesothelioma interest group. Journal of Thoracic Oncology. 2011;**6**:1304-1312

[39] Rintoul RC, Ritchie AJ, Edwards JG, et al. Efficacy and cost of video-assisted thoracoscopic partial pleurectomy versus talc pleurodesis in patients with malignant pleural mesothelioma (MesoVATS): An open-label, randomised controlled trial. Lancet. 2014;**384**:1118-1127

[40] Van Schil PE, Baas P, Gafaar R, et al. Trimodality therapy for malignant pleural mesothelioma: Results from an EORTC phase II multicentre trial. Eur Resp J. 2010;**36**:1362-1369

[41] Krug LM, Pass HI, Rusch VW, et al. Multicenter phase II trial of neoadjuvant pemetrexed plus cisplatin followed by extrapleural pneumonectomy and radiation for malignant pleural mesothelioma. Journal of Clinical Oncology. 2009;**27**:3007-3013

[42] Treasure T, Lang-Lazdunski L, Waller D, et al. Extra-pleural pneumonectomy versus no extra-pleural pneumonectomy for patients with malignant pleural mesothelioma: Clinical outcomes of the mesothelioma and radical surgery (MARS) randomised feasibility study. The Lancet Oncology. 2011;**12**:763-772

[43] Cao CQ, Yan TD, Bannon PG, McCaughan BC. A systematic review of extrapleural pneumonectomy for malignant pleural mesothelioma. Journal of Thoracic Oncology. 2010;**5**:1692-1703

Section 2

Clinical and Therapeutics

Chapter 2

Peritoneal Mesothelioma: Clinical and Therapeutic Aspects

Cristian Mesina, Mihaela-Iustina Mesina-Botoran, Theodor Viorel Dumitrescu, Mihai Calin Ciorbagiu and Cosmin Vasile Obleaga

Abstract

Mesothelioma is a very rare malignant disease that originates from mesothelial cells that line the serosa: pleura, peritoneum, pericardium, or testicular vaginal tunic. Peritoneal mesothelioma accounts for 7–10% of all mesotheliomas diagnosed, and ranks second after pleural localization of mesothelioma. The incidence of peritoneal mesothelioma is 0.5–3 cases per million in men and 0.2–2 cases per million in women. Diagnosis of peritoneal mesothelioma is difficult due to non-specific symptoms and because of this patients present in advanced stages of the disease. Histologically there are three major categories of malignant peritoneal mesothelioma: epithelioid, sarcomatoid, and biphasic. The differential diagnosis of peritoneal mesothelioma is made with peritoneal pseudomyxoma, ovarian tumors, and peritoneal metastases from colorectal cancer. An important role in differential diagnosis, in addition to immunohistochemistry, is played by various tumor markers and genetic tests. The treatment of peritoneal mesothelioma is performed by cytoreductive surgery (CRS) with hyperthermic intraperitoneal chemotherapy (HIPEC), with good results for patients in the early stages of the disease. For patients with advanced disease, a new treatment has been proposed: pressurized intraperitoneal aerosol chemotherapy (PIPAC). For patients who cannot use CRS and HIPEC, the only therapeutic option remains chemotherapy (systemic + intraperitoneal).

Keywords: peritoneal mesothelioma, cytoreductive surgery, hyperthermic intraperitoneal chemotherapy

1. Introduction

Mesotheliomas arise from cells lining the serosa: pleural, pericardial, peritoneal, and testicular vaginal tunic. Mesothelial tumors range from localized malignant mesothelioma to aggressive diffuse malignancies that invade the anatomical structures of the neighborhood and can give distant metastases. Rare mesothelial tumors that represent less than 1% of all diagnosed mesothelial tumors are paratesticular mesothelioma and pericardial mesothelioma. The peritoneal localization of mesothelioma is on the second place after the pleural localization. Peritoneal mesothelioma (PM) is a rare disease with an incidence of 0.6–3 per million in men and 0.2–2 per million in women [1]. Diffuse malignant peritoneal mesothelioma (DMPM), which accounts for 30% of all malignant mesotheliomas, is characterized by symptomatic polymorphism and difficulty in establishing a positive diagnosis. In this sense, the immunohistochemical examination has a very important role in differentiating this disease from peritoneal carcinomatosis [2].

2. Peritoneal mesothelioma: Symptomatology, histopathology, differential diagnosis, and treatment

2.1 Symptomatology of PM

The vast majority of patients are asymptomatic. The most common signs appear when the tumor mass compresses the neighboring organs or the rupture of cystic tumor formations mimicking the symptoms of acute peritonitis, as happened in the case operated and treated in our surgery clinic. Thus, the most common symptoms are abdominal pain, ascites, anorexia, weight loss, palpable tumor formation, and localized or generalized muscle defense [3].

Due to the more frequent localization of peritoneal mesothelioma on the pelvic peritoneum, peritoneal adhesions appear on the rectum, uterus, and bladder, causing the appearance of other symptoms such as dysuria, urinary symptoms, intestinal obstruction, and dyspareunia.

Peritoneal mesothelioma should be differentiated from multicystic peritoneal mesothelioma (MCPM) which is a benign, multicystic abdominal tumor such as cystic lymphangioma, endometriosis, cystic adenomatoid tumor, pseudomyxoma peritonei, and malignant peritoneal mesothelioma. For the positive diagnosis of MCPM, it is necessary to perform an immunohistochemical examination [3].

Benign multicystic peritoneal mesothelioma (BMPM) known as multilocular peritoneal cysts is an extremely rare disease which has the peritoneal mesothelium as a starting point. Although this disease is considered benign, relapse after surgery is reported in over 50% of cases [4] and two cases of malignant transformation have been reported [5]. Pathogenesis of the disease is unknown. There is a discussion of a possible etiopathogenicity related to pelvic inflammatory disease, Mediterranean fever, endometriosis, and a history of abdominal surgery. Three hypotheses have been proposed in the etiology of BMPM disease. One hypothesis argues that BMPM arises from an inflammatory process involving peritoneum, which results in hyperplastic and dysplastic reactive transformation of peritoneal mesothelial cells. Another theory supports the primary neoplastic origin without the involvement of a chronic inflammatory process. Other authors support the hormonal theory in which the development and progression of BMPM is closely related to sensitivity to sexual hormones. This theory is supported by the fact that BMPM has a higher incidence in women during the reproductive period and that BMPM responds to tamoxifen and gonadotropin-releasing hormone analogs [6]. Most authors agree on the fact that chronic peritoneal inflammatory process causes proliferation and migration of peripheral mesothelial cells often associated with metaplasia of the underlying connective tissue [6–8]. Transition between multicystic mesothelioma and adenomatoid tumor has been observed on several occasions [9, 10].

The symptoms of BMPM are insignificant but become apparent when the cystic tumors are large enough to produce mass effect on surrounding organs, or if the cysts break and produce an acute peritonitis-like reaction, as we have shown. Symptoms may be chronic abdominal and/or pelvic pain, abdominal distension, intestinal obstruction, and intestinal transit disorders [1, 11–13].

The physical examination may reveal muscle defense, abdominal distension, or acute appendicitis-like symptoms [14].

There are benign or malignant diseases that can mime BMPM. These diseases are intestinal lymphangioma and malignant peritoneal mesothelioma. Lymphangioma can be diagnosed when the cysts contain predominantly chyli fluid [15] and when the presence of lymphoid aggregates, smooth muscle cells, and D2-40-positive immunoexpression is discovered in the immunohistochemical examination. Malignant peritoneal mesothelioma has a history of asbestos exposure, abdominal pain, and weight loss.

2.2 Histopathology of PM

Three histological types of peritoneal mesothelioma have been described: epithelioid, sarcomatoid, and biphasic. Patients with sarcomatoid and biphasic subtypes have a more reserved prognosis than patients with the epithelioid subtype. Multicystic mesothelioma and well-differentiated papillary mesothelioma are forms of peritoneal mesothelioma that have a favorable prognosis.

2.2.1 Benign mesothelioma

Benign mesothelioma is a term applied to solitary lesions of peritoneum. Two types of benign mesothelial proliferation in the peritoneal cavity are benign multicystic peritoneal mesothelioma (MCPM) and adenomatoid tumor.

2.2.2 Malignant mesothelioma

Malignant mesothelioma is commonly found in adults and serum levels of osteopontin and mesothelin are serum biomarkers used for diagnosis.

Well-differentiated papillary mesothelioma of peritoneum is multicentric, extensive, and is characterized by prominent formation of papillae lined by bland mesothelial cell with minimal or no invasion. These are associated with an evolution without clinical symptoms, and people with this clinical form of mesothelioma have a long survival.

Deciduoid mesothelioma is characterized by the presence of large tumor cells with an abundant ground-glass cytoplasm that simulates the appearance of decidual cells. This histological form has been described in young women, located not only in the pelviperitoneal cavity but also in the pleural cavity in patients of both sexes. It is characterized by a short survival.

Mesothelioma with clear cell features can be confused with metastatic carcinoma from the kidney. The cytoplasmic clearing is due to the accumulation of glycogen in which case the alternative term glycogen-rich mesothelioma has been used.

Malignant mesothelioma with small cell is characterized by the presence of small cells. Most of reported cases have been immunoreactive for keratin and mesothelial markers including calretinin, CK 5/6, WT1, and podoplanin; some cases also stained for neuron-specific enolase and occasionally CD 57.

Lymphohistiocytoid mesothelioma is characterized microscopically by a diffuse proliferation of atypical histiocyte-like malignant mesothelial cells admixed with numerous lymphocytes (T-cell type) and lesser number of plasma cells. The phenotype of the histiocyte-like elements reflects their mesothelial nature and the behavior of this tumor is aggressive.

Pleomorphic mesothelioma in the WHO classification scheme is considered a variant of epithelioid mesothelioma and is characterized by pleomorphic large cells with abundant eosinophilic cytoplasm and single or multiple nuclei with marked variation in size and large nucleoli. The staining for traditional markers of mesothelioma-like calretinin, CK 5/6, and WT1 is variable but they are intense positive for pankeratin and cytokeratin 7. These tumors are a variant of sarcomatous tumors rather than epithelioid mesothelioma, being characterized by an aggressive behavior characteristic of sarcomatous tumors.

Desmoplastic mesothelioma is a subtype of sarcomatoid epithelioma, characterized by abundant deposition of fibrous tissue demonstrating a storiform arrangement of neoplastic spindle cells. The main differential diagnosis is with benign fibrous proliferations. Immunohistochemical receptors for keratin, calretinin, and WT1 is in favor of desmoplastic mesothelioma.

2.3 Role of immunohistochemistry, electron microscopy, and molecular testing in differential diagnosis of mesothelioma

2.3.1 Immunohistochemistry and electron microscopy

The diagnosis of malignant mesothelioma in the absence of detectable invasion is problematic in the absence of invasive disease. Homozygous deletion of $p16^{INK4a}$ (CDKN2A) detected using a fluorescent in situ hybridization (FISH) assay and loss of BAP1 expression by immunohistochemistry may be helpful in separating benign from malignant mesothelial proliferations including desmoplastic mesothelioma.

Other immunostains such as epithelial membrane antigen (EMA), p53, GLUT1, and IMP3 are proposed for separating benign from malignant mesothelial proliferations. Malignant epithelioid mesotheliomas need to be distinguished from metastatic carcinoma, specially adenocarcinomas with pseudo-mesotheliomatous growth pattern [3, 16].

The role of immunohistochemistry is in separating sarcomatoid mesotheliomas from sarcomatoid carcinomas and soft tissue sarcomas [2]. Mesotheliomas usually produce large amounts of hyaluronic acid, which can be demonstrated with the alcian blue or colloidal iron stains. The presence of obvious droplets of mucicarmine-positive or periodic acid-Schiff (PAS)-positive material in the cytoplasm of the tumor cell makes the diagnosis of mesothelioma very unlikely, although it does not rule it out completely inasmuch as the existence of rare mucin-positive mesotheliomas has been demonstrated.

Electron microscopy played an important role in the differential diagnosis between mesothelioma and metastatic carcinoma. This was primarily based on the appearance of the microvilli in the apical surface of the tumor cells, which in mesothelioma are longer and more slender than those in adenocarcinoma.

Many metastatic adenocarcinomas likely to be confused with mesothelioma are positive for cytokeratin 7, as are epithelioid mesotheliomas, making cytokeratin 7, as are epithelioid mesotheliomas, making cytokeratin 7 and 20 of limited value except in very specific context of metastases from the gastrointestinal tract.

The following immunostains are most commonly available and utilized in differential diagnosis of mesothelioma:

1. Epithelial markers that are usually present in both tumors (mesothelioma and metastatic carcinoma): pankeratins, EMA, and basement membrane components;

2. Organ-associated and lineage-specific markers that are often expressed in metastatic carcinoma but not mesothelioma: napsin A (lung and kidney), PAX8 (kidney, mullerian, thymus), CDX2 (gastrointestinal tract, pancreatobiliary),

p63/p40 (squamous cell, urothelial), and GATA3 (breast, urothelial, squamous cell);

3. Markers that are usually expressed in metastatic carcinoma but not mesothelioma: MOC-31, Ber-EP4, carcinoembryonic antigen (CEA), B72.3, BG8, CD15, MUC4, and claudiu-4;

4. Markers that are usually expressed in mesothelioma but not in carcinoma: calretinin (breast, mullerian serous), WT1 (breast, mullerian serous), keratin 5/6 (urothelial, squamous cell), D2-40/podoplanin (mullerian serous, squamous cell), and thrombomodulin (squamous cell).

2.3.2 Molecular genetic features

Mutations in the TP 53 gene are uncommon. In 60–80% of mesothelioma cases, homozygous deletion of $p16^{INK4a}$ (CDKN2A) is found, which is an investigation used to differentiate benign mesothelial disorders from malignant mesothelial proliferations. CDKN2A deletion is a potential biomarker for a more aggressive course in some cases of mesothelioma. The most common recurrent somatic mutations in malignant mesothelioma target three genes functioning as tumor suppressors: cyclin-dependent kinase inhibitor 2A (CDKN2A), BCRA1-associated protein 1 (BAP1), and neurofibromin 2 (merlin) (NF2).

2.3.3 Differential radiological and histopathological diagnosis

Differential diagnosis is made with other peritoneal malignancies such as peritoneal pseudomyxoma, ovarian tumors, and peritoneal metastases from colorectal cancer. Peritoneal pseudomyxoma is a rare disease characterized by multifocal epithelial deposits in the peritoneal cavity, secreted by mucin, with or without gelatinous ascites, in the absence of extraperitoneal involvement [17]. It was first described by Werth and later by Rokitansky in 1942, being considered a fatal condition, with unexplained etiology. It predominates in women, the ovarian tumor pathology being incriminated as responsible in a significant percentage in the etiopathogenesis of peritoneal pseudomyxoma. In men, adenoma (mucocele) appendicular tumors and appendicular adenocarcinoma are the main cause described [17]. Virtually any primary solid tumor is the epicenter of the malignancy. In the case of peritoneal pseudomixoma, the predominant tumor volume is in the peritoneum, and the primary tumor is insignificant, whether it is appendicular, ovarian, or in other organs [18]. Pseudomyxoma peritonei involves the presence of mucinous, gelatinous deposits in the peritoneum, deposits that can reach impressive sizes. Thus, death can be caused by respiratory failure. It seems that the basis of this condition is a certain type of mucous cells that have a special pattern—the presence of MUC2 [18]. Removal of the tumor and gelatinous material is the purpose of treatment.

Peritoneal pseudomixoma is the most serious complication of the appendicular mucocele and develops as a result of spontaneous or iatrogenic implantation of the tumor into the peritoneal cavity [19]. The peritoneal and occasionally pleural pseudomixoma, which appeared as a result of the evolution of the appendicular mucocele, is rare and constitutes 6–8.8% [19–21]. Pseudomucinous cysts of the ovary, usually associated with appendicular mucocele, are the predominant cause of peritoneal pseudomixoma in older women and in men; the origin of peritoneal pseudomixoma is usually the vermicular appendix [21]. The pathology has a slow evolution through the loss of intestinal function, fistula formation, and eventual death. The most common complications are occlusion and intestinal bleeding.

Extra-abdominal eruption of appendicular cystadenocarcinoma with spontaneous cutaneous fistula formation is extremely rare, being published only four cases in the world literature [22–25]. The pathogenetic mechanism of spontaneous skin fistula formation in patients with mucinous cystadenocarcinoma of the appendix is enigmatic, but we assume that the occurrence of this complication depends on the malignant nature of the tumor.

Patients with appendicular mucocele are asymptomatic in about 25% of cases; even in the case of large lesions, the most common complaints are pain in the right iliac fossa, similar to acute appendicitis and palpable tumor formation in 50% of cases [20, 21].

2.4 Treatment

Malignant peritoneal mesothelioma (MPM) is a rare disease with a recurrence rate of 40–50% after surgical debulking. Identifying the histological type of peritoneal mesothelioma, the number of invaded lymph nodes, and the Ki-67 proliferation marker are very important parameters for surgical treatment, but this is possible in most cases after laparotomy and cytoreductive surgery (CRS). The preoperative CT scan, performed by an experienced radiologist, can help us identify anatomical sites unfavorable for surgical treatment such as intestinal serosa and/or porta hepatis [26].

2.4.1 Cytoreductive surgery (CRS)

For the selection of patients benefiting from CRS, the peritoneal cancer index (PCI) is used, which consists of combining a score [27] given by 13 abdomino-pelvic regions (central, right upper, epigastrium, upper left, left flank, left lower, pelvis, right lower, right flank, upper jejunum, lower jejunum, upper ileum, lower ileum) to which lesion size score is added (LS 0—no tumor seen; LS 1—tumor up to 0.5 cm; LS 2—tumor up to 5 cm, and LS 3—tumor >5 cm or confluence).

In MPM, there is an intraoperative extensive invasion at the level of the parietal and visceral peritoneum on the surface of the small and large intestines but also in the mesentery and mesocolon. Lymph nodes will be removed whenever there is a suspicion of invasion, but a complete CRS may require resections of the small and large intestines (especially the splenic angle of the colon or the sigmoid colon). In order to achieve HIPEC, a complete hemostasis is needed; otherwise, intraperitoneal hemorrhage occurs during the procedure. Before HIPEC, an extensive intraoperative peritoneal toilet will be performed either with distilled water or with diluted hydrogen peroxide (0.25%) or povidone iodine, which aim at the mechanical cleansing of possible cancer cells.

Recently, the use of cytoreductive surgery (CRS) in the treatment of peritoneal mesothelioma with hyperthermic intraperitoneal chemotherapy (HIPEC) has been discussed [28]. Median overall survival for patients with peritoneal mesothelioma treated by CRS and HIPEC ranges from 29 to 95 months [29–32].

Research [29] on 405 patients with peritoneal mesothelioma from 29 centers in Europe and the US reported that after treatment of peritoneal mesothelioma with CRS and HIPEC, a median survival of 53 months and 5-year overall survival rate of 47%. Overall survival of patients with peritoneal mesothelioma treated with chemotherapy alone (pemetrexed + cisplatin) was poor (approximately 13 months).

A study [33] of 1514 patients with peritoneal mesothelioma who were treated with CRS, CRS and HIPEC, and chemotherapy alone showed a survival of 52 months for CRS, 61 months for CRS and HIPEC, and 17 months after chemotherapy.

The reduction of the MPM recurrence rate was obtained by combining CRS with HIPEC. The study conducted by Nizri and colleagues [34] on 19 patients with MPM who underwent CRS combined with HIPEC showed that after a median follow-up of 69 months, all patients were alive and only 4 of the 19 patients had recurrences (21%).

2.4.2 Hyperthermic intraperitoneal chemotherapy (HIPEC), early postoperative intraperitoneal chemotherapy (EPIC), pressurized intraperitoneal aerosol chemotherapy (PIPAC), and normothermic intraperitoneal chemotherapy (NIPEC) in treatment of MPM

Additional chemotherapy was used to treat patients with MPM according to three therapeutic protocols as follows:

1. HIPEC with doxorubicin and cisplatin

2. Early postoperative intraperitoneal chemotherapy (EPIC) with paclitaxel that was added intraperitoneally in the first 5 days after CRS.

3. HIPEC then EPIC and then long-term intraperitoneal paclitaxel or pemetrexed intraperitoneally to which cisplatin is added intravenously as an adjunct to normothermic intraperitoneal chemotherapy (NIPEC).

In the absence of CRS and HIPEC, the median survival of patients with MPM is approximately 1 year. Aggressively applied surgical treatment along with additional chemotherapy increased the median survival of patients with MPM over 5 years.

The standard recommendations for HIPEC are cisplatin if renal function is good (250 mg/m^2), cisplatin plus doxorubicin, cisplatin plus mitomycin, or mitomycin only. There are also authors who use bidirectional chemotherapy by adding systemic ifosfamide plus mesna disulfide by continuing the 90-minute infusion of HIPEC with doxorubicin and cisplatin.

Survival in patients with MPM is improved in patients who used CRS plus HIPEC compared to patients who used CRS plus hyperthermic perioperative chemotherapy.

Recent studies [35] suggest a new therapeutic modality for patients with peritoneal mesothelioma: pressurized intraperitoneal aerosol chemotherapy (PIPAC). This new therapeutic modality, combined with systemic chemotherapy, may be an option for patients to whom CRS and HIPEC cannot be applied.

A retrospective study [36] of 29 patients with peritoneal mesothelioma treated with PIPAC (doxorubicin + cisplatin) showed encouraging results. Many patients with advanced peritoneal mesothelioma do not benefit from CRS and HIPEC, where chemotherapy (systemic + intraperitoneal) remains the only therapeutic option.

2.4.3 Molecular therapy and immunotherapy

One hope for molecular therapy in patients with MPM was the identification of ALK rearrangements that would be present in 3% of patients with MPM. This has been shown to be present in patients <40 years of age who have not been exposed to asbestos fibers. It is hoped that these patients will benefit from ALK inhibitors.

Gefitinib and erlotinib, which are tyrosine kinase inhibitors, acting on the epidermal growth factor receptor (EGFR), have been shown to have no significant action in MPM. By contrast, angiokinase inhibitors (nintedanib) acting on VEGF receptors, platelet-derived-growth factors, fibroblastic growth factors, and Src and Abl kinase signaling improved progression-free survival in patients with MPM when co-administered with pemetrexed and cisplatin [37].

Bevacizumab, which is an anti-VEGF antibody [38] in combination with cisplatin and pemetrexed, significantly increased overall survival in patients with MPM. Immune checkpoint inhibitors such as anti-CTLA 4 (tremelimumab and iplimumab) and anti-PD1 antibodies (avelumab and durvalumab) are under investigation.

2.4.4 Recommendations in the treatment of MPM

The recommendations discussed at the Washington DC 2016 meeting by the Peritoneal Surface Oncology Group International (PSOGI) regarding therapeutic strategies [39] in patients with MPM were the following:

1. Patients with MPM who are operable will be given CRS and HIPEC. The applied surgical treatment will include peritonectomy procedures (there are still controversies related to parietal peritonectomy: selective parietal peritonectomy vs. complete parietal peritonectomy). During the surgical treatment, it will be taken into account that the preservation of the viscera is preferred and the invaded retroperitoneal lymph nodes will be removed. Optimal cytoreduction will be assessed by validated peritoneal staging scoring systems: CC or R-score, in which the CRS objectives are to achieve a CC-0 or CC-1 score, in which the peritoneal nodules have a diameter of less than 2.5 mm.
   HIPEC will be used with cisplatin and carboplatin, either alone or in combination with doxorubicin, pemetrexed, ifosfamide, and mitomycin. Mitomycin has also been used as the only chemotherapeutic agent but with a slight decrease in survival. Normothermic intraperitoneal chemotherapy with pemetrexed and other chemotherapeutic agents has also been used with a slight increase in the survival of patients with MPM.

2. Patients with well-differentiated papillary and multicystic mesothelioma will be treated with either CRS alone or HIPEC-associated CRS depending on the stage of the disease. The benefit of combining HIPEC therapy is unknown.

3. Patients with biphasic, sarcomatoid, or unresectable PMP will only be treated by systemic chemotherapy. New chemotherapeutic agents are being tested, especially for patients who have seen an increase in Ki67, seen in immunohistochemical studies.

4. The contribution of adjuvant chemotherapy to the treatment of patients with PMP is unknown. The study conducted by Sugarbaker and colleagues in 2017 [27] on long-term adjuvant combined intraperitoneal and systemic chemotherapy showed promising results.
   It has been shown in published studies that the response rate of malignant epithelioid mesothelioma to systemic chemotherapy is around 20%. The chemotherapeutic agents used are pemetrexed, carboplatin, cisplatin, and bevacizumab.

5. New chemotherapeutic agents such as anti-mesothelin antibody (anetumumab), anti-PDL-1 (pembrolizumab), CAR T cells, and *Listeria*-based immunotherapy can improve the survival of patients with PMP.

There are still no clear recommendations in the follow-up of patients with MPM after radical excision surgery [40]. There is a follow-up guide developed by the European Society for Medical Oncology for pleural mesothelioma, but no frequency or methods of investigation used in the postoperative period (CT, MRI, or ultra-sonography) are specified. Serum follow-up markers are conventional: CA125 and mesothelin.

2.5 Conclusions

Patients with peritoneal mesothelioma, due to nonspecific symptoms, present in advanced stages of the disease. An important role in determining the histological subtype of peritoneal mesothelioma is played by immunohistochemistry. Multidisciplinary management is preferred for patients with MPM. CRS and HIPEC appear to be the most effective therapeutic modalities in the treatment of MPM. Bidirectional chemotherapy is able to increase the resectability rate in patients with diffuse MPM, initially considered unresectable. Modern therapies such as molecular therapy and immunotherapy can increase the overall survival of patients with MPM. New therapeutic approaches have improved the prognosis only for patients in the early stages of the disease.

Conflict of interest

The authors declare no conflict of interest.

Abbreviations

DMPM	diffuse malignant peritoneal mesothelioma
MCPM	multicystic peritoneal mesothelioma
BMPM	benign multicystic peritoneal mesothelioma
PM	peritoneal mesothelioma
MPM	malignant peritoneal mesothelioma
CRS	cytoreductive surgery
PSOGI	Peritoneal Surface Oncology Group International
HIPEC	hyperthermic intraperitoneal chemotherapy
PIPAC	pressurized intraperitoneal aerosol chemotherapy
EPIC	early postoperative intraperitoneal chemotherapy
NIPEC	normothermic intraperitoneal chemotherapy
PCI	peritoneal cancer index
EGFR	epidermal growth factor receptor

Author details

Cristian Mesina[1*], Mihaela-Iustina Mesina-Botoran[2], Theodor Viorel Dumitrescu[1], Mihai Calin Ciorbagiu[1] and Cosmin Vasile Obleaga[1]

1 Department of Surgery, Emergency County Hospital of Craiova, University of Medicine and Pharmacy of Craiova, Craiova, Romania

2 Department of Human Anatomy, University of Medicine and Pharmacy of Craiova, Craiova, Romania

*Address all correspondence to: mesina.cristian@doctor.co

References

[1] Boffetta P. Epidemiology of peritoneal mesothelioma: A review. Annals of Oncology. 2007;**18**:985-990

[2] Meşină C, Vasile I, Vîlcea ID, Pasalega M, Parvanescu H, et al. Sarcoamele de părți moi--probleme de diagnostic şi tratament [Soft tissue sarcoma--Problems of diagnosis and treatment]. Chirurgia (Bucur). 2010;**105**(2):257-266

[3] Meşină C, Dumitrescu TV, Mogoantă SŞ, Ciorbagiu MC, Cristian DA, et al. An unusual cause of acute surgical abdomen: Benign multicystic peritoneal mesothelioma associated with adenomatous tumor. Romanian Journal of Morphology and Embryology. 2018;**59**(3):971-976

[4] Vyas D, Pihl K, Kavuturu S, Vyas A. Mesothelioma as a rapidly developing giant abdominal cyst. World Journal of Surgical Oncology. 2012;**10**:277-281

[5] González-Moreno S, Yan H, Alcorn KW, Sugarbaker PH. Malignant transformation of "benign" cystic mesothelioma of the peritoneum. Journal of Surgical Oncology. 2002;**79**(4):243-251

[6] Occhionorelli S, Tartarini D, Pascale G, Maccatrozzo S, Stano R, Vasquez G. Benign multicystic mesothelioma of peritoneum complicating acute appendicitis in a man: A case report. Journal of Medical Case Reports. 2016;**10**(2):44-46

[7] Momeni M, Pereira E, Grigoryan G, Zakashansky K. Multicystic benign cystic mesothelioma presenting as a pelvic mass. Case Reports in Obstetrics and Gynecology. 2014;**2014**:852483

[8] Oks M, He T, Palkar A, Esposito MJ, Koenig SJ. Benign multicystic mesothelioma causing bilateral pneumothoraces. Annals of the American Thoracic Society. 2015;**12**(7):1106-1109

[9] Chan JKC, Fong MH. Composite multicystic mesothelioma and adenomatoid tumor of the uterus: Different morphological manifestations of the same process? Histopathology. 1996;**29**(4):375-377

[10] Livingstone EG, Guis MS, Pearl ML, Stern JL, Brescia RJ. Diffuse adenomatoid tumor of the uterus with a serosal papillary cystic component. International Journal of Gynecological Pathology. 1992;**11**(4):288-292

[11] Wang TB, Dai WG, Liu DW, Shi HP, Dong WG. Diagnosis and treatment of benign multicystic peritoneal mesothelioma. World Journal of Gastroenterology. 2013;**19**(39):6689-6692

[12] Safioleas MC, Constantinos K, Michael S, Konstantinos G, Constantinos S, Alkiviadis K. Benign multicystic peritoneal mesothelioma: A case report and review of the literature. World Journal of Gastroenterology. 2006;**12**(35):5739-5742

[13] Mesina C, Vasile I, Vilcea ID, Pasalega M, Calota F, Enache DS, et al. Carcinoid tumors of the appendix: Problems of diagnosis and treatment. Chirurgia (Bucur). 2011;**106**(2):239-245

[14] Khuri S, Gilshtein H, Abboud W, Assalia A, Kluger Y. Benign cystic mesothelioma of the peritoneum: A rare case and review of the literature. Case Reports in Oncology. 2012;**5**(3):667-670

[15] Meşină C, Paşalega M, Calotă F, Comănescu V, Vîlcea D, et al. Limfangiomul intestinal hemoragic – prezentare de caz. Chirurgia (Bucur). 2006;**101**(2):201-204

[16] Meşină C, Stoean CL, Stoean R, Dumitrescu TV, Mogoanta SS, et al.

Immunohistochemical evaluation of tumor budding in colorectal cancer: An important parameter with prognostic value. Romanian Journal of Morphology and Embryology. 2019;**60**(3):841-846

[17] van Ruth S, Hart AA, Bonfrer JM, Verwaal VJ, Zoetmulder FA. Prognostic value of baseline and serial carcinoembryonic antigen and carbohydrate antigen 19.9 measurements in patients with pseudomyxoma peritonei treated with cytoreduction and hyperthermic intraperitoneal chemotherapy. Department of Surgical Oncology, The Netherlands Cancer Institute/Antoni van Leeuwenhoek Hospital, Amsterdam, The Netherlands. Annals of Surgical Oncology. 2002;**9**(10):961-967

[18] O'Connell JT, Tomlinson JS, Roberts AA, McGonigle KF, Barsky SH. Pseudomyxoma peritonei is a disease of MUC2-expressing goblet cells. The American Journal of Pathology. 2002;**161**(2):551-564

[19] Minni F, Petrella M, Morgani A, Santini D, Marrano D. Giant mucocele of the appendix. Diseases of the Colon and Rectum. 2001;**44**:1034

[20] Landen S, Bertrand C, Maddern GJ, Herman D, Pourbaix A, De Neve A, et al. Appendiceal mucoceles and pseudomyxoma peritonei. Surgery, Gynecology & Obstetrics. 1992;**175**:401

[21] Fann JI, Vierra M, Fisher D, Oberhelman HA Jr, Cobb L. Pseudomyxoma peritonei. Surgery, Gynecology & Obstetrics. 1993;**177**:441

[22] Arly KS, Stephenson DV Jr, Davis WC. Giant retroperitoneal mucocele simulating pseudomyxoma peritonei and mucinous adenocarcinoma. American Journal of Surgery. 1968;**116**:439

[23] Nishitani K, Nishitani H, Shimoda Y. Cutaneous invasion of mucinous adenocarcinoma of the appendix. The Journal of Dermatology. 1987;**14**:167

[24] Koizumi J, Noguchi H. Pseudomyxoma retroperitonei with spontaneous skin fistula. Abdominal Imaging. 1999;**24**:193

[25] Nakao A, Sato S, Nakashima A, Nabeyama A, Tanaka N. Appendiceal mucocele of mucinous cystadenocarcinoma with a cutaneous fistula. The Journal of International Medical Research. 2002;**30**:452

[26] Chandramohan A, Thrower A, Smith SA, Shah N, Moran B. A method for communicating radiological extent of peritoneal malignancy. Clinical Radiology. 2017;**72**:972-980

[27] Sugarbaker PH, Chang D. Long-term regional chemotherapy for patients with epithelial malignant peritoneal mesothelioma results in improved survival. European Journal of Surgical Oncology. 2017;**43**(7):1228-1235

[28] Gilani SNS, Mehta A, Garcia-Fadrique A, Rowaiye B, Jenei V, Dayal S, et al. Outcomes of cytoreductive surgery with hyperthermic intraperitoneal chemotherapy for peritoneal mesothelioma and predictors of survival. International Journal of Hyperthermia. 2018;**34**:578-584

[29] Yan TD, Deraco M, Elias D, Glehen O, Levine EA, Moran BJ, et al. A novel tumor-node-metastasis (TNM) staging system of diffuse malignant peritoneal mesothelioma using outcome analysis of a multi-institutional database*. Cancer. 2011;**117**:1855-1863

[30] Helm JH, Miura JT, Glenn JA, Marcus RK, Larrieux G, Jayakrishnan TT, et al. Cytoreductive surgery and hyperthermic intraperitoneal chemotherapy for malignant peritoneal mesothelioma: A systematic review and meta-analysis.

Annals of Surgical Oncology. 2015;**22**:1686-1693

[31] Alexander HR Jr, Bartlett DL, Pingpank JF, Libutti SK, Royal R, Hughes MS, et al. Treatment factors associated with long-term survival after cytoreductive surgery and regional chemotherapy for patients with malignant peritoneal mesothelioma. Surgery. 2013;**153**:779-786

[32] Baratti D, Kusamura S, Cabras AD, Bertulli R, Hutanu I, Deraco M. Diffuse malignant peritoneal mesothelioma: Long-term survival with complete cytoreductive surgery followed by hyperthermic intraperitoneal chemotherapy (HIPEC). European Journal of Cancer. 2013;**49**:3140-3148

[33] Verma V, Sleightholm RL, Rusthoven CG, Koshy M, Sher DJ, Grover S, et al. Malignant peritoneal mesothelioma: National practice patterns, outcomes, and predictors of survival. Annals of Surgical Oncology. 2018;**25**:2018-2026

[34] Nizri E, Baratti D, Guaglio M, et al. Multicystic mesothelioma: Operative and long-term outcomes with cytoreductive surgery and hyperthermic intra peritoneal chemotherapy. European Journal of Surgical Oncology. 2018;**44**(7):1100-1104. DOI: 10.1016/j.ejso.2018.03.004

[35] Alyami M, Hübner M, Grass F, Bakrin N, Villeneuve L, Laplace N, et al. Pressurised intraperitoneal aerosol chemotherapy: Rationale, evidence, and potential indications. The Lancet Oncology. 2019;**20**:e368-e377

[36] Giger-Pabst U, Demtröder C, Falkenstein TA, Ouaissi M, Götze TO, Rezniczek GA, et al. Pressurized intraperitoneal aerosol chemotherapy (PIPAC) for the treatment of malignant mesothelioma. BMC Cancer. 2018;**18**:442

[37] Grosso F, Steele N, Novello S, et al. Nintedanib plus pemetrexed/cisplatin in patients with malignant pleural mesothelioma: Phase II results from the randomized, placebo-controlled LUME-Meso Trial. Journal of Clinical Oncology. 2017;**35**:3591-3600

[38] Zalcman G, Mazieres J, Margery J, et al. Bevacizumab for newly diagnosed pleural mesothelioma in the Mesothelioma Avastin Cisplatin Pemetrexed Study (MAPS): A randomised, controlled, open-label, phase 3 trial. Lancet. 2016;**387**:1405-1414

[39] Turaga KK, Deraco M, Alexander HR. Current management strategies for peritoneal mesothelioma. International Journal of Hyperthermia. 2017;**33**(5):579-581. DOI: 10.1080/02656736.2017.1320591

[40] Habbel VSA, Mahler EA, Feyerabend B, Oldhafer KJ, Lipp MJ. Das diffuse maligne peritoneale Mesotheliom (DMPM) – eine seltene Diagnose [Diffuse malignant peritoneal mesothelioma (DMPM) - A rare diagnosis]. Zeitschrift für Gastroenterologie. 2020;**58**(2):146-151. DOI: 10.1055/a-1083-6962

Chapter 3

Current Mesothelioma Treatment and Future Perspectives

Danijela Štrbac, Katja Goričar, Viljem Kovač and Vita Dolžan

Abstract

The established treatments in malignant mesothelioma are based on trimodality approach including surgery, radiation and chemotherapy. Such approach has proved to clinically benefit mesothelioma patients, however the current treatments seem to have reached a limit regarding the survival and disease control. One approach to overcome the limitations of current treatments is focused on finding appropriate serum or genetic biomarkers that could support personalized medicine and improve outcomes with established treatment modalities in mesothelioma patients. The other approach is exploiting better understanding of molecular and genetic characteristics of mesothelioma to search for new treatment modalities. Immunotherapy with anti PD-1, PD-L1 and CTLA-4 agents is a new frontier in mesothelioma treatment. As in many solid tumors, CAR-T cell therapy is emerging from the field of hematological malignancies. Immunomodulatory approaches seem to be a new perspective in treatment of malignant mesothelioma. This chapter aims to explore possible new therapeutic approaches in mesothelioma.

Keywords: mesothelioma treatment, genetic biomarkers, patient based therapy, gene therapy, immunomodulation

1. Introduction: trimodality approach to mesothelioma treatment

The established treatments in mesothelioma are based on trimodality approach including surgery, radiation and chemotherapy. Such concept for MM was introduced in the late 1990s by Sugarbaker et al. It was proposed that the treatment of mesothelioma should start with extrapleural pneumonectomy (EPP) and followed by chemoradiation [1]. A study of 120 patients concluded that a 40% survival rate was feasible in patients with epithelial histology and negative nodes. A need for a more precise staging and more effective management strategies was stated [1].

Two and a half decades after the trimodality approach was introduced, little has changed in the treatment of mesothelioma. According to the National Comprehensive Cancer Network (NCCN) guidelines, in stages I to III of surgically operable mesothelioma, a chemotherapy regimen of pemetrexed with cisplatin or carboplatin is proposed in either preoperative or postoperative setting. For patients who received the entire trimodality approach, a median survival of 20 to 29 months has been reported [2, 3].

However, the majority of mesothelioma patients are diagnosed in advanced stages, are inoperable and/or have a poor performance (WHO performance status (PS) of 2 or above). Treatment with systemic chemotherapy significantly improves survival of MM patients and patients are usually treated with a platinum agent in combination with either pemetrexed or gemcitabine [4, 5]. Studies have shown that both chemotherapy regimens have comparable results [4, 6, 7]. The only FDA approved treatment for advanced stages of mesothelioma is pemeterexed/cisplatin with possible options of vinorelbine or gemcitabine.

The combination with pemetrexed has become standard treatment in various clinical guidelines such as the NCCN, the European Society of Medical Oncology (ESMO) and American Society of Clinical Oncology (ASCO) [3, 8, 9]. In a Slovenian clinical study, gemcitabine in a prolonged infusion with cisplatin was shown as one of the most successful systemic treatments [4, 6]. Although current treatments clinically benefit mesothelioma patients, they seem to have reached a limit regarding the survival and disease control. One approach to overcome the limitations of current treatments is focused on finding appropriate serum or genetic biomarkers that could support personalized medicine and improve outcomes with established treatment modalities in mesothelioma patients [10].

A deeper understanding of tumor biology has also enabled the development of target drugs. These drugs target and inhibit the molecular signaling pathways along which a tumor develops, grows, and spreads. Several target drugs have been tested in the treatment of MM in the last few years, but so far no targeted treatment has shown sufficient results to allow patients to be treated outside of clinical trials. Slovenian researchers also participated in one of these clinical trials with target drugs, focusing on bortezomib and cisplatin treatment [11]. The addition of bevacizumab to gemcitabine and cisplatin or pemetrexed and cisplatin has shown slightly better results. An addition of bevacizumab to the pemetrexed/cisplatin doublet has increased overall survival for up to 2.7 months, but it is suitable only for patients that do not have bleeding tendencies or a risk of thrombosis. Bevacizumab treatment has shown sufficiently promising results that it has come into routine use in the United States [12].

Among the novel treatment approaches, immunotherapy is becoming the most promising, especially with immune checkpoint inhibitors such as inhibitors of programmed cell death 1 (PD-1, *PDCD1*) and programmed cell death 1 ligand 1 (PD-L1, *CD274*) [13]. Based on the results of clinical trials, it is currently estimated that 20–25% of patients with MM may benefit from treatment with immune checkpoint inhibitors [14].

Subsequent treatment lines are less effective in mesothelioma. Novel second line treatment approaches include immunotherapy with PD-1 inhibitors, such as pembrolizumab or nivolumab. Nivolumab can be used in a combination with CTLA-4 inhibitor, ipilimumab [15, 16]. However, if immunotherapy is not accessible or has a high toxicity such as pneumonitis, a chemotherapy regimen with gemcitabine or vinorelbine is a valid option.

The aim of this chapter is to explore possible new therapeutic approaches in mesothelioma.

2. Biomarker guided chemotherapy treatment in malignant mesothelioma

Research of biomarkers in malignant mesothelioma has been ongoing for the last twenty years. Predictive and prognostic biomarkers are also needed to support the treatment and follow up of patients with MM [17]. It has been shown that apart from clinical characteristics such as C-reactive protein or tumor stage, serum and genetic markers may be associated with treatment outcome in MM [10, 18–29]. Traditional research in mesothelioma biomarkers involves soluble molecules, such as mesothelin, fibulin and survivin [18, 20, 30], but novel serum biomarkers for disease risk, diagnosis and treatment are also emerging [31]. Mesothelin is the only clinically validated biomarker in the diagnosis of mesothelioma. However, there are no predictive biomarkers that would allow patient stratification and a more personalized treatment approach. Studies have shown that patient stratification based on genetic biomarkers could improve chemotherapy outcome, but these approaches are not routinely used in the clinic yet [32, 33]. It is becoming more and more widely accepted that pharmacogenomics is enabling personalized medicine by testing for genetic variability in drug metabolizing enzymes, transporters, and drug targets thus accounting for interindividual variability in drug levels (pharmacokinetics), drug response (pharmacodynamics) and adverse events. Using pharmacogenomics approach, the treatment of malignant mesothelioma could perhaps be tailored also to individual's genetic make-up, thereby promising safer and also more effective drug treatment [34–38].

2.1 Pharmacogenomics of cisplatin treatment

Cytotoxic activity of cisplatin and other platinum analogues is based on their ability to covalently bind to DNA, form intrastrand DNA adducts or interstrand cross-links, and lead to replication and transcription arrest. DNA adducts are recognized and repaired by nucleotide excision repair (NER) mechanisms. Genetic variability in NER genes such as ERCC excision repair 2 (*ERCC2*) and ERCC excision repair 1 (*ERCC1*) was associated with malignant mesothelioma treatment outcomes [23, 39]. In particular, *ERCC1* rs3212986 (c.*197G > T) wild-type genotype was significantly associated with better progression-free survival (PFS), but also with increased odds of treatment-related toxicities. The risk for cisplatin toxicity was also increased in patients with wild type genotype of *ERCC2* rs1799793 (p.Asn312Asp) polymorphism [23].

Interstrand crosslinks are among the most detrimental forms of DNA damage because both DNA strands are affected. As translesion DNA polymerases are needed to bypass these crosslinks and restore one of the two DNA strands in order for repair mechanisms to proceed, they may also contribute to response to cisplatin treatment [40]. Studies have shown that disruption or suppression of expression of two genes participating in translesion repair, *REV3L* and *REV1* modifies sensitivity to cisplatin [41, 42]. Similarly, *REV3L* polymorphisms rs465646 (c.*461C > T) and rs462779 (p. Thr1224Ile) were significantly associated with longer overall survival in MM patients treated with cisplatin based doublet chemotherapy, while *REV1* rs3087403 (p. Val138Met) allele and *REV1* TGT haplotype were associated with increased risk for leukopenia and neutropenia [43].

2.2 Pharmacogenomics of pemetrexed treatment

Only a few studies investigated the influence of genetic polymorphism in the folate metabolic pathways on treatment outcome in MM patients that received antifolate chemotherapeutic pemetrexed [22, 44, 45]. MM patients with at least one polymorphic *MTHFD1* rs2236225 (p.Arg653Gln) allele had a lower response rate and shorter PFS than carriers of two wild-type alleles. Furthermore, polymorphisms in pemetrexed transporter genes, such as *ABCC2* and *SLCO1B1* influenced the risk for toxicity in patients receiving antifolates [22]. Another study investigating 5,10-methylenetetrahydrofolate reductase (*MTHFR*) and *ERCC1* gene polymorphisms failed to prove an association between the selected polymorphisms and treatment outcome, but did show that a 6-base pair insertion/deletion in the 3′ untranslated region of the thymidylate synthase *TS* gene was associated with differences in disease control rate and PFS in MM [44].

2.3 Pharmacogenomics of gemcitabine treatment

Because gemcitabine is frequently used in combination with cisplatin in Slovenian mesothelioma patients, a study investigating pharmacogenomics factors that may influence the response to gemcitabine has also been performed. Deoxycytidine kinase and ribonucleotide reductase M1 (*RRM1*) were investigated as the main metabolic and target enzymes, respectively. The study indicated that the *RRM1* rs1042927 (c.*316C > A) polymorphism significantly decreased overall survival. Two promoter polymorphisms, *RRM1* rs11030918 (c.-524 T > C) and rs12806698 (c.-37C > A), decreased the odds of nausea and vomiting, while the *RRM1* TTCCA haplotype was associated with worse tumor response and worse overall survival [25]. DNA repair gene polymorphisms, particularly *XRCC1* rs25487 (p.Arg399Gln), may also modify the response to gemcitabine/platinum combination chemotherapy and effect overall survival in mesothelioma patients [24].

2.4 Clinical-pharmacogenomic models predicting outcome of malignant mesothelioma treatment

Pharmacogenomic findings motivated further research into developing a clinical-pharmacogenomic model combining clinical and genetic data and an algorithm that would enable treatment stratification in MM. The clinical-pharmacogenomic model that could help predict response to gemcitabine/cisplatin combination and survival of MM patients included C-reactive protein, histological type, performance status, *RRM1* rs1042927, *ERCC2* rs13181, *ERCC1* rs3212986, and *XRCC1* rs25487. The clinical-pharmacogenomic model that could help predict response to pemetrexed/cisplatin combination included C-reactive protein, *MTHFD1* rs2236225, and *ABCC2* rs2273697 [10]. An algorithm for treatment stratification was proposed based on both clinical-pharmacogenomic models, where a more favorable chemotherapy regimen could be recommended in 64.2% of patients: pemetrexed/cisplatin in 35.9% and gemcitabine/cisplatin in 28.3%. The algorithm predicted that 21.4% of patients would respond equally well to both treatments, but 14.5% of patients would probably not respond well to either [10]. The algorithm requires further independent validation, before it could be used in the clinical decision making, but is nevertheless proof that a tailored treatment could be applied in mesothelioma chemotherapy.

3. Future perspectives in the treatment of mesothelioma

3.1 Immunotherapy in mesothelioma

Immunotherapeutic approach is proposed as second line treatment in mesothelioma. It entails three basic immunological targets as either anti-PD-1 (nivolumab, pembrolizumab), anti-PD-L1 (atezolizumab, durvalumab) or anti-CTLA-4 (ipilimumab) or in combination, such as nivolumab/ipilimumab. The most promising trial data come from a combination of ipilimumab and nivolumab with median survival of 15.9 months. However, there is 94% rate of treatment related adverse events with combination immunotherapy [15].

Therefore, monotherapy approaches have been proposed in second line setting. Pembrolizumab in monotherapy is promising with a 20% partial response rate with a median response duration of one year. Grade 3 or 4 toxicity rate is reported at 20% [46, 47].

These data, however promising, present a high rate of toxicity and rather limited response and survival rates. With analogy to the genetic biomarkers for cytotoxic chemotherapy, further research should be done to determine genetic biomarkers in immunotherapy [48].

3.2 Gene therapy in mesothelioma

The principle of gene therapy is to infiltrate tumor cells and deactivate genes involved in tumor growth and progression. Classical example of gene therapy is to target p53 expression and induce apoptosis in mesothelioma cells. Several clinical trials targeted crucial pathways in mesothelioma cells that would ultimately lead to cell death using oncolytic viruses as vectors. The genes injected in these trials were interleukin-2, interferon α2b, herpes simplex virus thymidine kinase, and interferon β. The response was achieved mostly around the injected site in the pleural cavity, however some clinical response was noted months after injection into tumor site. The direct cell death that was the goal of this gene therapy was limited, however a delayed immune response was proposed since several antibodies were found in patients with response to treatment [49].

While gene therapy with oncolytic viruses as vectors of injection has been tested as monotherapy, combination with chemotherapy has been proposed to achieve a dual effect of local and systemic disease control [50–53].

3.3 CAR-T cells in mesothelioma

Chimeric antigen receptors (CARs) are genetically encoded artificial fusion molecules that can re-program the specificity of peripheral blood polyclonal T-cells against a selected cell surface target. The overall structure of a CAR consists of four domains joined in series, namely: an antigen recognition domain (targeting moiety), a hinge/spacer, a transmembrane element and a signaling endodomain. The CAR ectodomain determines target specificity and, most commonly, contains elements derived from a monoclonal antibody [54].

Unparalleled clinical efficacy has recently been demonstrated using this approach to treat patients with refractory B-cell malignancy, such as lymphomas. Solid tumors were the next to be included in CAR T cell (CAR-T) immunotherapy, but have posed certain toxicity challenges, such as on target off tumor toxicity. A fatal toxicity was noted in human epidermal growth factor receptor 2 (HER-2) CAR-T cells which led to respiratory and multi organ failure with cytokine release syndrome [55].

Also mesothelioma has been studied in the setting of CAR-T therapy. An *in vitro* study of MET receptor tyrosine kinase specific CAR-T cells was designed to target MET expressing mesothelioma cells. The data from the *in vivo* animal models showed that this type of CAR therapy can be safe and effective in MET expressing mesothelioma [56]. A small study reported two patients treated with mesothelin targeting CAR-T cells (CAR-T meso cells). The investigators in this study used a novel approach of mRNA engineered CAR-T cells to overcome the off- tumor on target toxicity. They concluded that the treatment with CAR-T meso cells is feasible in pretreated patients with progressive disease, since they reported partial tumor response [57].

4. Conclusions

The treatment of mesothelioma presents a clinical challenge, especially in the second and further lines of treatment. There is still place for improvement of current treatment strategies, in particular the response to chemotherapy, by enabling pharmacogenomics based informed selection of patients who would benefit most from a particular treatment regimen. Based on our previous studies, clinical-pharmacogenomic prediction models and algorithms could facilitate treatment stratification and contribute to improved treatment outcome in MM. The future of mesothelioma treatment seems to involve immunologically based treatment with either the already present immunotherapy or the evolving CAR-T therapy. The innovation of the decades old principles of CAR-T cell therapy has proven to be successful in hematological malignancies and mesothelioma seems to be on the forefront of research in solid tumors with such innovations as are the mRNA CAR-T meso cells.

Acknowledgements

This work was financially supported by the Slovenian Research Agency (ARRS Grants No. P1-0170, P3-0307, L3-8203 and L3-2622).

Conflict of interest

The authors declare no conflict of interest.

Author details

Danijela Štrbac[1], Katja Goričar[2], Viljem Kovač[1] and Vita Dolžan[2]*

1 Institute of Oncology Ljubljana, Ljubljana, Slovenia

2 Pharmacogenetics Laboratory, Institute of Biochemistry, Faculty of Medicine, University of Ljubljana, Ljubljana, Slovenia

*Address all correspondence to: vita.dolzan@mf.uni-lj.si

References

[1] Sugarbaker DJ, Heher EC, Lee TH, Couper G, Mentzer S, Corson JM, et al. Extrapleural pneumonectomy, chemotherapy, and radiotherapy in the treatment of diffuse malignant pleural mesothelioma. Journal of Thoracic and Cardiovascular Surgery. 1991;102(1): 10-14; discussion 14-15.

[2] Katirtzoglou N, Gkiozos I, Makrilia N, Tsaroucha E, Rapti A, Stratakos G, et al. Carboplatin plus pemetrexed as first-line treatment of patients with malignant pleural mesothelioma: a phase II study. Clinical Lung Cancer. 2010;11(1):30-35. DOI: 10.3816/CLC.2010.n.005

[3] Ettinger DS, Wood DE, Akerley W, Bazhenova LA, Borghaei H, Camidge DR, et al. NCCN Guidelines Insights: Malignant Pleural Mesothelioma, Version 3.2016. Journal of the National Comprehensive Cancer Network. 2016;14(7):825-836. DOI: 10.6004/jnccn.2016.0087

[4] Kovac V, Zwitter M, Zagar T. Improved survival after introduction of chemotherapy for malignant pleural mesothelioma in Slovenia: Population-based survey of 444 patients. Radiology and Oncology. 2012;46(2):136-144. DOI: 10.2478/v10019-012-0032-0

[5] Damhuis RA, Schroten C, Burgers JA. Population-based survival for malignant mesothelioma after introduction of novel chemotherapy. European Respiratory Journal. 2012;40(1):185-189. DOI: 10.1183/09031936.00153611

[6] Kovac V, Zwitter M, Rajer M, Marin A, Debeljak A, Smrdel U, et al. A phase II trial of low-dose gemcitabine in a prolonged infusion and cisplatin for malignant pleural mesothelioma. Anti-Cancer Drugs. 2012;23(2):230-238. DOI: 10.1097/CAD.0b013e32834d7a1c

[7] Lee CW, Murray N, Anderson H, Rao SC, Bishop W. Outcomes with first-line platinum-based combination chemotherapy for malignant pleural mesothelioma: a review of practice in British Columbia. Lung Cancer. 2009;64(3):308-313. DOI: 10.1016/j.lungcan.2008.09.008

[8] Baas P, Fennell D, Kerr KM, Van Schil PE, Haas RL, Peters S, et al. Malignant pleural mesothelioma: ESMO Clinical Practice Guidelines for diagnosis, treatment and follow-up. Annals of Oncology. 2015;26 Suppl 5:v31-39. DOI: 10.1093/annonc/mdv199

[9] Kindler HL, Ismaila N, Armato SG, 3rd, Bueno R, Hesdorffer M, Jahan T, et al. Treatment of Malignant Pleural Mesothelioma: American Society of Clinical Oncology Clinical Practice Guideline. Journal of Clinical Oncology. 2018;36(13):1343-1373. DOI: 10.1200/JCO.2017.76.6394

[10] Goricar K, Kovac V, Dolzan V. Clinical-pharmacogenetic models for personalized cancer treatment: application to malignant mesothelioma. Scientific Reports. 2017;7:46537. DOI: 10.1038/srep46537

[11] O'Brien ME, Gaafar RM, Popat S, Grossi F, Price A, Talbot DC, et al. Phase II study of first-line bortezomib and cisplatin in malignant pleural mesothelioma and prospective validation of progression free survival rate as a primary end-point for mesothelioma clinical trials (European Organisation for Research and Treatment of Cancer 08052). European Journal of Cancer. 2013;49(13):2815-2822. DOI: 10.1016/j.ejca.2013.05.008

[12] Zalcman G, Mazieres J, Margery J, Greillier L, Audigier-Valette C, Moro-Sibilot D, et al. Bevacizumab for newly diagnosed pleural mesothelioma in the Mesothelioma

Avastin Cisplatin Pemetrexed Study (MAPS): a randomised, controlled, open-label, phase 3 trial. Lancet. 2016;387(10026):1405-1414. DOI: 10.1016/s0140-6736(15)01238-6

[13] Tazzari M, Brich S, Tuccitto A, Bozzi F, Beretta V, Spagnuolo RD, et al. Complex Immune Contextures Characterise Malignant Peritoneal Mesothelioma: Loss of Adaptive Immunological Signature in the More Aggressive Histological Types. Journal of Immunology Research. 2018;2018:5804230. DOI: 10.1155/2018/5804230

[14] Dozier J, Zheng H, Adusumilli PS. Immunotherapy for malignant pleural mesothelioma: current status and future directions. Translational Lung Cancer Research. 2017;6(3):315-324. DOI: 10.21037/tlcr.2017.05.02

[15] Disselhorst MJ, Quispel-Janssen J, Lalezari F, Monkhorst K, de Vries JF, van der Noort V, et al. Ipilimumab and nivolumab in the treatment of recurrent malignant pleural mesothelioma (INITIATE): results of a prospective, single-arm, phase 2 trial. The Lancet Respiratory Medicine. 2019;7(3):260-270. DOI: 10.1016/S2213-2600(18)30420-X

[16] Scherpereel A, Mazieres J, Greillier L, Lantuejoul S, Do P, Bylicki O, et al. Nivolumab or nivolumab plus ipilimumab in patients with relapsed malignant pleural mesothelioma (IFCT-1501 MAPS2): a multicentre, open-label, randomised, non-comparative, phase 2 trial. The Lancet Oncology. 2019;20(2):239-253. DOI: 10.1016/S1470-2045(18)30765-4

[17] Carbone M, Adusumilli PS, Alexander HR, Jr., Baas P, Bardelli F, Bononi A, et al. Mesothelioma: Scientific clues for prevention, diagnosis, and therapy. CA: A Cancer Journal for Clinicians. 2019;69(5):402-429. DOI: 10.3322/caac.21572

[18] Kovac V, Dodic-Fikfak M, Arneric N, Dolzan V, Franko A. Fibulin-3 as a biomarker of response to treatment in malignant mesothelioma. Radiology and Oncology. 2015;49(3):279-285. DOI: 10.1515/raon-2015-0019

[19] Mineo TC, Ambrogi V. Malignant pleural mesothelioma: factors influencing the prognosis. Oncology (Williston Park). 2012;26(12):1164-1175.

[20] Goricar K, Kovac V, Dodic-Fikfak M, Dolzan V, Franko A. Evaluation of soluble mesothelin-related peptides and MSLN genetic variability in asbestos-related diseases. Radiology and Oncology. 2020;54(1):86-95. DOI: 10.2478/raon-2020-0011

[21] Goricar K, Kovac V, Franko A, Dodic-Fikfak M, Dolzan V. Serum Survivin Levels and Outcome of Chemotherapy in Patients with Malignant Mesothelioma. Disease Markers. 2015;2015:316739. DOI: 10.1155/2015/316739

[22] Goricar K, Kovac V, Dolzan V. Polymorphisms in folate pathway and pemetrexed treatment outcome in patients with malignant pleural mesothelioma. Radiology and Oncology. 2014;48(2):163-172. DOI: 10.2478/raon-2013-0086

[23] Erčulj N, Kovač V, Hmeljak J, Dolžan V. The influence of platinum pathway polymorphisms on the outcome in patients with malignant mesothelioma. Annals of Oncology. 2011;23:961-967. DOI: 10.1093/annonc/mdr324

[24] Erculj N, Kovac V, Hmeljak J, Franko A, Dodic-Fikfak M, Dolzan V. DNA repair polymorphisms and treatment outcomes of patients with

malignant mesothelioma treated with gemcitabine-platinum combination chemotherapy. Journal of Thoracic Oncology. 2012;7(10):1609-1617. DOI: 10.1097/JTO.0b013e3182653d31

[25] Erculj N, Kovac V, Hmeljak J, Franko A, Dodic-Fikfak M, Dolzan V. The influence of gemcitabine pathway polymorphisms on treatment outcome in patients with malignant mesothelioma. Pharmacogenetics and Genomics. 2012;22(1):58-68. DOI: 10.1097/FPC.0b013e32834e3572

[26] Fontana V, Vigani A, Pistillo MP, Giannoni U, Rosemberg I, Canessa PA, et al. The Correlation of Serum Mesothelin Level With Pleural Thickness in Malignant Pleural Mesothelioma Makes it a Valuable Tool for Monitoring Tumor Progression. Journal of Thoracic Oncology. 2019;14(5):e92-e94. DOI: 10.1016/j.jtho.2018.12.026

[27] Arnold DT, De Fonseka D, Hamilton FW, Rahman NM, Maskell NA. Prognostication and monitoring of mesothelioma using biomarkers: a systematic review. British Journal of Cancer. 2017;116(6):731-741. DOI: 10.1038/bjc.2017.22

[28] Creaney J, Robinson BWS. Malignant Mesothelioma Biomarkers: From Discovery to Use in Clinical Practice for Diagnosis, Monitoring, Screening, and Treatment. Chest. 2017;152(1):143-149. DOI: 10.1016/j.chest.2016.12.004

[29] Hoda MA, Dong Y, Rozsas A, Klikovits T, Laszlo V, Ghanim B, et al. Circulating activin A is a novel prognostic biomarker in malignant pleural mesothelioma - A multi-institutional study. European Journal of Cancer. 2016;63:64-73. DOI: 10.1016/j.ejca.2016.04.018

[30] Hmeljak J, Erculj N, Dolzan V, Pizem J, Kern I, Kovac V, et al. Is survivin expression prognostic or predictive in malignant pleural mesothelioma? Virchows Archiv. 2013;462(3):315-321. DOI: 10.1007/s00428-013-1373-9

[31] Strbac D, Goricar K, Dolzan V, Kovac V. Matrix Metalloproteinases Polymorphisms as Baseline Risk Predictors in Malignant Pleural Mesothelioma. Radiology and Oncology. 2018;52(2):160-166. DOI: 10.2478/raon-2018-0005

[32] Simon GR, Schell MJ, Begum M, Kim J, Chiappori A, Haura E, et al. Preliminary indication of survival benefit from ERCC1 and RRM1-tailored chemotherapy in patients with advanced nonsmall cell lung cancer: evidence from an individual patient analysis. Cancer. 2012;118(9):2525-2531. DOI: 10.1002/cncr.26522

[33] Mazzoni F, Cecere FL, Meoni G, Giuliani C, Boni L, Camerini A, et al. Phase II trial of customized first line chemotherapy according to ERCC1 and RRM1 SNPs in patients with advanced non-small-cell lung cancer. Lung Cancer. 2013;82(2):288-293. DOI: 10.1016/j.lungcan.2013.08.018

[34] Relling MV, Evans WE. Pharmacogenomics in the clinic. Nature. 2015;526(7573):343-350. DOI: 10.1038/nature15817

[35] Pirmohamed M. Personalized pharmacogenomics: predicting efficacy and adverse drug reactions. Annual Review of Genomics and Human Genetics. 2014;15:349-370. DOI: 10.1146/annurev-genom-090413-025419

[36] Relling MV, Klein TE. CPIC: Clinical Pharmacogenetics Implementation Consortium of the Pharmacogenomics Research Network. Clinical Pharmacology and Therapeutics. 2011;89(3):464-467. DOI: 10.1038/clpt.2010.279

[37] Dunnenberger HM, Crews KR, Hoffman JM, Caudle KE, Broeckel U, Howard SC, et al. Preemptive clinical pharmacogenetics implementation: current programs in five US medical centers. Annual Review of Pharmacology and Toxicology. 2015;55:89-106. DOI: 10.1146/annurev-pharmtox-010814-124835

[38] Peterson JF, Roden DM, Orlando LA, Ramirez AH, Mensah GA, Williams MS. Building evidence and measuring clinical outcomes for genomic medicine. Lancet. 2019;394(10198):604-610. DOI: 10.1016/s0140-6736(19)31278-4

[39] Ting S, Mairinger FD, Hager T, Welter S, Eberhardt WE, Wohlschlaeger J, et al. ERCC1, MLH1, MSH2, MSH6, and βIII-tubulin: resistance proteins associated with response and outcome to platinum-based chemotherapy in malignant pleural mesothelioma. Clinical Lung Cancer. 2013;14(5):558-567.e553. DOI: 10.1016/j.cllc.2013.04.013

[40] Makridakis NM, Reichardt JK. Translesion DNA polymerases and cancer. Frontiers in Genetics. 2012;3:174. DOI: 10.3389/fgene.2012.00174

[41] Lin X, Okuda T, Trang J, Howell SB. Human REV1 modulates the cytotoxicity and mutagenicity of cisplatin in human ovarian carcinoma cells. Molecular Pharmacology. 2006;69(5):1748-1754. DOI: 10.1124/mol.105.020446

[42] Doles J, Oliver TG, Cameron ER, Hsu G, Jacks T, Walker GC, et al. Suppression of Rev3, the catalytic subunit of Pol{zeta}, sensitizes drug-resistant lung tumors to chemotherapy. Proceedings of the National Academy of Sciences of the United States of America. 2010;107(48):20786-20791. DOI: 10.1073/pnas.1011409107

[43] Goricar K, Kovac V, Dolzan V. Polymorphisms in translesion polymerase genes influence treatment outcome in malignant mesothelioma. Pharmacogenomics. 2014;15(7):941-950. DOI: 10.2217/pgs.14.14

[44] Powrozek T, Kowalski DM, Krawczyk P, Ramlau R, Kucharczyk T, Kalinka-Warzocha E, et al. Correlation between TS, MTHFR, and ERCC1 gene polymorphisms and the efficacy of platinum in combination with pemetrexed first-line chemotherapy in mesothelioma patients. Clinical Lung Cancer. 2014;15(6):455-465. DOI: 10.1016/j.cllc.2014.06.009

[45] Zucali PA, Giovannetti E, Destro A, Mencoboni M, Ceresoli GL, Gianoncelli L, et al. Thymidylate synthase and excision repair cross-complementing group-1 as predictors of responsiveness in mesothelioma patients treated with pemetrexed/carboplatin. Clinical Cancer Research. 2011;17(8):2581-2590. DOI: 10.1158/1078-0432.CCR-10-2873

[46] Alley EW, Lopez J, Santoro A, Morosky A, Saraf S, Piperdi B, et al. Clinical safety and activity of pembrolizumab in patients with malignant pleural mesothelioma (KEYNOTE-028): preliminary results from a non-randomised, open-label, phase 1b trial. The Lancet Oncology. 2017;18(5):623-630. DOI: 10.1016/s1470-2045(17)30169-9

[47] Metaxas Y, Rivalland G, Mauti LA, Klingbiel D, Kao S, Schmid S, et al. Pembrolizumab as Palliative Immunotherapy in Malignant Pleural Mesothelioma. Journal of Thoracic Oncology. 2018;13(11):1784-1791. DOI: 10.1016/j.jtho.2018.08.007

[48] Goricar K, Kovac V, Dolzan V. The influence of PD-1 and PD-L1 polymorphisms on cisplatin-related toxicity in malignant mesothelioma (14th European ISSX Meeting). Accessed September 21, 2020. Available

at: http://issx.confex.com/issx/17euro/webprogram/Paper37441.html.

[49] Tada Y, Takiguchi Y, Hiroshima K, Shimada H, Ueyama T, Nakamura M, et al. Gene therapy for malignant pleural mesothelioma: present and future. Oncology Research. 2008;17(6):239-246. DOI: 10.3727/096504008786991602

[50] Tagawa M, Tada Y, Shimada H, Hiroshima K. Gene therapy for malignant mesothelioma: current prospects and challenges. Cancer Gene Therapy. 2013;20(3):150-156. DOI: 10.1038/cgt.2013.1

[51] Suveg K, Putora PM, Berghmans T, Glatzer M, Kovac V, Cihoric N. Current efforts in research of pleural mesothelioma-An analysis of the ClinicalTrials.gov registry. Lung Cancer. 2018;124:12-18. DOI: 10.1016/j.lungcan.2018.07.007

[52] Sterman DH, Kaiser LR, Albelda SM. Gene therapy for malignant pleural mesothelioma. Hematology/Oncology Clinics of North America. 1998;12(3):553-568. DOI: 10.1016/s0889-8588(05)70008-3

[53] Takagi-Kimura M, Yamano T, Tamamoto A, Okamura N, Okamura H, Hashimoto-Tamaoki T, et al. Enhanced antitumor efficacy of fiber-modified, midkine promoter-regulated oncolytic adenovirus in human malignant mesothelioma. Cancer Science. 2013;104(11):1433-1439. DOI: 10.1111/cas.12267

[54] Whilding LM, Maher J. CAR T-cell immunotherapy: The path from the by-road to the freeway? Molecular Oncology. 2015;9(10):1994-2018. DOI: 10.1016/j.molonc.2015.10.012

[55] Morgan RA, Yang JC, Kitano M, Dudley ME, Laurencot CM, Rosenberg SA. Case report of a serious adverse event following the administration of T cells transduced with a chimeric antigen receptor recognizing ERBB2. Molecular Therapy. 2010;18(4):843-851. DOI: 10.1038/mt.2010.24

[56] Thayaparan T, Petrovic RM, Achkova DY, Zabinski T, Davies DM, Klampatsa A, et al. CAR T-cell immunotherapy of MET-expressing malignant mesothelioma. Oncoimmunology. 2017;6(12):e1363137. DOI: 10.1080/2162402X.2017.1363137

[57] Beatty GL, Haas AR, Maus MV, Torigian DA, Soulen MC, Plesa G, et al. Mesothelin-specific chimeric antigen receptor mRNA-engineered T cells induce anti-tumor activity in solid malignancies. Cancer Immunology Research. 2014;2(2):112-120. DOI: 10.1158/2326-6066.CIR-13-0170

Section 3

Emerging Drugs

Chapter 4

Emerging Drug Therapies for Mesothelioma

Derek B. Oien, Jeremy Chien, Julian Molina and Viji Shridhar

Abstract

The systemic chemotherapy combination of cisplatin and pemetrexed has been the mesothelioma standard of care for well over a decade. This regimen has only achieved a disappointing overall median survival of about 1 year. Improved survival has been reported when systemic chemotherapy is combined with surgery and radiotherapy, and for using localized chemotherapy in some cases. The choice of mesothelioma treatment often depends on the anatomical location, histologic subtype, and disease progression. Several experimental drugs have also been investigated in mesothelioma, often with limited positive results that maintain the reputation of mesothelioma as a graveyard for drug development. This chapter will review the use of drug treatment in mesothelioma and highlight emerging experimental drug therapies in clinical trials. Experimental drugs for mesothelioma include inhibitors for checkpoints, epidermal growth factor, AXL, focal adhesion kinase, vascular endothelial growth factor, poly-ADP-ribose-polymerase, and hippo signaling.

Keywords: targeted drugs, experimental therapeutics, molecular therapies, drug combinations, NF2 mutations, BAP1 mutations

1. Introduction

The treatment of mesothelioma currently varies by primary origin of the tumor, histologic subtype, and disease progression. The most common mesothelioma is malignant pleural mesothelioma (about 80% of cases) [1]. Research for new drug treatments are often investigated in pleural mesothelioma and later extrapolated to less common types such as peritoneal mesothelioma (about 10% of cases). Both of these mesothelioma types have the same three subtypes of epithelioid, sarcomatoid, and biphasic histology. Biphasic mesothelioma is a combination of epithelioid and sarcomatoid histology, each contributing to at least 10% of the tissue [2]. Mesothelioma tends to spread regionally, then into the alternate thoracic lobe for pleural mesothelioma or across the abdomen for peritoneal mesothelioma, and can metastasize across the diaphragm or as distant metastases [2, 3]. Distant metastases were found in a postmortem study in over half of the 318 pleural mesothelioma patients examined, while distant metastasizes of peritoneal mesothelioma are not as common [2, 4]. Surgery is more common when disease is diagnosed early and tumors are resectable, but most patients are diagnosed at later stages of disease when they are not candidates. For pleural mesothelioma, extrapleural pneumonectomy and pleurectomy/decortication are the most common nonpalliative procedures for tumors that are confined to the excised region [5]. Some of these patients will be treated with postoperative radiation and systemic chemotherapy, while the benefits of preoperative treatment are still being investigated. For epithelioid peritoneal mesothelioma, cytoreductive surgery is often combined with perioperative chemotherapy [2]. Cytoreductive surgery has been found to have minimal benefit for sarcomatoid and biphasic peritoneal mesothelioma, and systemic chemotherapy is often the first line treatment for these patients [6]. Treatment for relapsed and treatment-refractory mesothelioma is generally palliative or experimental. Currently, there are about 200 initiated and active clinical trials for mesothelioma listed at clinicaltrials.gov (U.S. National Library of Medicine), and the majority of these are drug-based interventions.

There are no targeted therapies currently approved for mesothelioma. Many ongoing research studies and clinical trials are investigating receptor tyrosine kinase inhibitors and checkpoint inhibitors of the immune system. Surprisingly, very few studies are being done that specifically target frequent genetic alterations in mesothelioma. In this review, we discuss the current chemotherapy and highlight emerging experimental drugs for mesothelioma treatment.

2. Systemic and localized chemotherapy

The current chemotherapy standard of care for mesothelioma is a systemic combination of cisplatin and pemetrexed. Adding pemetrexed with cisplatin improved overall median survival of pleural mesothelioma patients from 9.3 months with cisplatin alone to 12.1 months for the combination, which was determined by a phase III clinical trial of the combination in 2003 [7]. Second-line treatments include cisplatin combined with gemcitabine or irinotecan [8–10], and vinorelbine monotherapy [11]. Depending on the disease progression, systemic chemotherapy is often combined with surgery or radiation. The prediction of which late-stage patients will benefit from surgery has proven to be difficult [5]. Radiotherapy alone has not been shown to improve overall survival, but this method is used in combination with surgery or systemic chemotherapy and for palliative purposes. Systemic cisplatin and pemetrexed therapy also remains the standard of care for peritoneal mesothelioma, and this regimen is often used for sarcomatoid and biphasic histologic subtypes [6]. Combining gemcitabine with cisplatin was reported to achieve an overall median survival of about 27 months for patients with unresectable peritoneal mesothelioma, but this combination has also shown considerable toxicity [9]. Similar to several other abdominal cancers, many epithelioid peritoneal mesothelioma patients benefit from intraperitoneal chemotherapy administration.

Cytoreductive surgery followed by perioperative hyperthermic (or heated, hot) intraperitoneal chemotherapy for epithelial peritoneal mesothelioma patients (about 75% of peritoneal mesothelioma patients [2]) has extended overall median survival, which was reported as 53 months [12] and 38 months [13] in two separate multi-institutional studies. The drugs are heated to 42°C and administered to the peritoneal cavity for hours, often while rocking the patient to improve drug dissemination [2]. Intraperitoneal administration of chemotherapy gained attention in the 1980s when this route was shown to have a superior pharmacokinetic profile for cisplatin over intravenous injection in canines [14]. With intraperitoneal administration, most of the chemotherapy remained in the peritoneal cavity and therefore much higher concentrations of drugs could be used, which were up to 30 times greater than common doses for intravenous injection [2, 15]. The effectiveness of hyperthermic intraperitoneal chemotherapy is based on the limits of drug penetration depth and correlates to the ability for achieving complete or near-complete cytoreduction [2, 16]. The drugs used are often varied combinations of cisplatin, mitomycin-C, and doxirubicin [6]. A significant proportion of patients have also benefited from additional long-term normothermic intraperitoneal chemotherapy following the hyperthermic perioperative dosing [6].

Overall, the main chemotherapy drugs for mesothelioma have led to unsatisfactory overall median survival percentages even when combined with radiation and surgical methods. Many mesothelioma patients try experimental drugs as part of clinical trials or compassionate-use programs. Unfortunately, mesothelioma has gained a reputation as a graveyard for drug development based on the minimal successes and modest extensions of overall survival from experimental drugs. Clinical trials to evaluate targeted drugs in mesothelioma tumors with specific genetic alterations have only recently increased to a relatively small number.

3. Frequent genetic alterations

The most well-known and frequent genetic alterations in mesothelioma are mutations in *BAP1*, *NF2*, and *TP53* genes and deletion of the *CDKN2A* gene. These mutations, along with mutations in *LATS2* and *SETD2*, were reported as the most frequent in two independent sequencing studies of mesothelioma tissues [17, 18]. Activation of the LATS2 kinase is regulated by NF2, and the SET2D protein is an H3 histone methyltransferase associated with tumor suppressor activity [19]. While the high frequency of some mutations in mesothelioma have been known for decades (e.g. *NF2*) and others have been discovered within the last decade (e.g. *BAP1*), there are still no targeted therapies approved for mesothelioma. Clinical trials requiring genetic testing for inclusion will be discussed in the next section.

Mutations in *BAP1*, the gene for the BRCA1-associated protein-1 deubiquitinating enzyme, were initially associated with mesothelioma as germline hereditary mutations [20], but it is now estimated that about 60% of mesothelioma tumors contain a mutation in *BAP1* (the majority being somatic acquired mutations) [5, 21–23]. It has been demonstrated that BAP1 regulates the DNA repair and apoptotic signaling in response to asbestos exposure [24, 25], which is the most common cause of mesothelioma. BAP1 loss also has been correlated to elevated trimethylation of H3 lysine 27 in mice, which recently lead to targeting the enhancer of zeste homolog 2 (EZH2) methyltransferase as a potential mesothelioma treatment strategy [26]. Germline *BAP1* mutations have been found in over 200 families across the globe, and about a third of cancer diagnoses in carriers of *BAP1* mutations are types of mesothelioma [5, 27]. BAP1-negative mesothelioma tumors mainly consist of the epithelioid histologic subtype [5].

The most unique frequent mutations for mesothelioma are that of the *NF2* gene. The *NF2* gene encodes the merlin protein (also known as neurofibromin 2), which has tumor suppressor activity and is associated with cell cycle/growth control through the hippo pathway [28]. Canonical hippo signaling controls the yes-associated protein (YAP), a transcription regulator for many cell cycle-associated genes. Verteporfin is a small molecule with YAP inhibitor activity that is approved for macular degeneration and has recently shown activity against *in vitro* mesothelioma models [29, 30]. We have found that mesothelioma cells are very sensitive to the antimalarial drug quinacrine *in vitro* when inactivating *NF2* mutations are present (*unpublished data*). While there are no clinical trials for mesothelioma involving these molecules, both of these drugs have potential to be repurposed for NF2-negative mesothelioma. Outside of mesothelioma, *NF2* mutations are only frequently found in a few rare neurological cancers and the inherited neurofibromatosis type II syndrome. It is estimated that about 40% of mesothelioma tumors have *NF2* mutations, although there are many other hippo-related genes found mutated in mesothelioma tumors at lower frequencies [31, 32].

Inactivation of the *TP53* and *CDKN2A* genes are not unique to mesothelioma, and these genes are known to be the first- and second-most common mutations in all cancer, respectively. The *TP53* gene is only mutated in about 15% of mesothelioma tumors [18], far below the *TP53* mutation rate for most other cancer types. Deletion of the *CDKN2A* gene is found in about 45% of all mesothelioma tumors [18]. The *CDKN2A* (cyclin-dependent kinase inhibitor 2A) gene encodes for p14arf and p16INK4a tumor suppressor proteins that regulate cell cycle activities.

Mansfield and colleagues recently used mate-pair sequencing analyses to show most mesothelioma tumors contain several chromosomal rearrangements [33]. In 22 mesothelioma patient samples examined, 13 samples contained *CDKN2A* deletions and 14 samples had *NF2* deletions. This suggests the genetics of mesothelioma cancer cells may be altered more than previously detected in several studies that used next generation sequencing methods.

4. Emerging molecular therapies

Pemetrexed was the last drug to be approved by the FDA for mesothelioma in 2004, and now several novel molecular therapies which have had success in other cancers are now being tried in mesothelioma. Among the long list, angiogenesis inhibitors and immune checkpoint inhibitors have arguably made the most progress in clinical trials.

In a recent phase III clinical trial, the vascular endothelial growth factor (VEGF) inhibitor bevacizumab was added to cisplatin and pemetrexed combination therapy for patients with unresectable mesothelioma (**Table 1**, NCT00651456) [34]. This three-drug combination resulted in significant improvement for overall survival to 18.8 months without a significant negative impact for health-related quality-of-life in patients with advanced pleural mesothelioma [35]. This combination has not yet been approved by the FDA. Another VEGF inhibitor, cediranib, was evaluated in combination with cisplatin and pemetrexed in a phase II trial for unresectable, chemotherapy naïve pleural mesothelioma (NCT01064648). This study reported improved progression-free survival and response rate, but further development has been halted based on the toxicity profile obtained during the trial [36]. Two other multitarget drugs that inhibit VEGF receptors, axitinib and nintedanib, did not meet clinical benefit goals when combined with cisplatin and pemetrexed [37]. Axitinib was unsuccessful when evaluated in a phase II trial for chemotherapy naïve, unresectable epithelioid pleural mesothelioma (NCT01211275). Combining nintedanib with pemetrexed and cisplatin did not meet the primary progression-free survival goals in a phase III clinical trial for advanced pleural mesothelioma [38]. The European-based BEAT-mesophase III trial is in the early stages and adds atezolizumab to the cisplatin, pemetrexed, and bevacizumab combination for advanced pleural mesothelioma (NCT03762018). Atezolizumab is a monoclonal antibody against programmed cell death-ligand 1 (PD-L1). The MiST phase II trial also has an arm for evaluating atezolizumab and bevacizumab in relapsed mesothelioma that has positive PD-L1 expression (NCT03654833). It is estimated that up to 25% of mesothelioma patients may benefit from immune checkpoint inhibitors [5].

Interest in PD-L1 inhibitors for mesothelioma is based on prior success of these inhibitors in other cancer types and a study showing about 40% of the 212 mesothelioma patient samples examined express PD-L1 [17]. It was also shown in the latter study that high PD-L1 expression correlated with poor survival for the mesothelioma patients. In addition to the BEAT-meso clinical trial, atezolizumab is also being evaluated in a phase II trial on unresectable or advanced pleural mesothelioma (NCT03786419). The combination of PD-L1 inhibitor durvalumab with cisplatin

Study title	Drug interventions	Phase	NCT number
Mesothelioma Avastin Plus Pemetrexed-cisplatin Study*	Bevacizumab, pemetrexed, cisplatin	2/3	NCT00651456
Pemetrexed Disodium and Cisplatin With or Without Cediranib Maleate in Treating Patients With Malignant Pleural Mesothelioma	Cediranib, pemetrexed, cisplatin	2	NCT01064648
Standard Chemotherapy With or Without Axitinib in Malignant Mesothelioma (N08CPA)*	Axitinib, pemetrexed, cisplatin	2	NCT01211275
Nintedanib (BIBF 1120) in Mesothelioma**	Nintedanib, pemetrexed, cisplatin	2/3	NCT01907100
Bevacizumab and Atezolizumab in Malignant Pleural Mesothelioma (BEAT-meso)	Bevacizumab, atezolizumab, cisplatin, pemetrexed	3	NCT03762018
Mesothelioma Stratified Therapy (MiST): A Multi-drug Phase II Trial in Malignant Mesothelioma	Bemcentinib & pembrolizumab, atezolizumab & bevacizumab, rucaparib, abemaciclib	2	NCT03654833
A Study of Atezolizumab in Unresectable or Advanced Malignant Pleural Mesothelioma	Atezolizumab	2	NCT03786419
Pembrolizumab in Patients With Advanced Malignant Pleural Mesothelioma	Pembrolizumab, pemetrexed, cisplatin	2/3	NCT02784171
CheckpOiNt Blockade For Inhibition of Relapsed Mesothelioma	Nivolumab	3	NCT03063450
Study of Nivolumab Combined With Ipilimumab Versus Pemetrexed and Cisplatin or Carboplatin as First Line Therapy in Unresectable Pleural Mesothelioma Patients	Nivolumab, ipilimumab, pemetrexed, cisplatin, carboplatin	3	NCT02899299
Randomized, Double-blind Study Comparing Tremelimumab to Placebo in Subjects With Unresectable Malignant Mesothelioma	Tremelimumab	2	NCT01843374
A Phase 2 Study of Durvalumab in Combination With Tremelimumab in Malignant Pleural Mesothelioma**	Tremelimumab, durvalumab	2	NCT03075527
Pembrolizumab + Defactinib In Pleural Mesothelioma	Pembrolizumab, defactinib	1	NCT04201145
Targeted Therapy Directed by Genetic Testing in Treating Patients With Advanced Refractory Solid Tumors, Lymphomas, or Multiple Myeloma (The MATCH Screening Trial)	Several targeted drugs including defactinib for tumors with NF2 inactivating mutations	2	NCT02465060
Everolimus (RAD001) for the Treatment of Malignant Pleural Mesothelioma With Merlin/NF2 Loss as a Biomarker to Predict Sensitivity*	Everolimus	2	NCT01024946
Study of the EZH2 Inhibitor Tazemetostat in Malignant Mesothelioma*	Tazemetostat	2	NCT02860286
A Trial of Niraparib in BAP1 and Other DNA Damage Response (DDR) Deficient Neoplasms (UF-STO-ETI-001)	Niraparib	2	NCT03207347
Olaparib in People With Malignant Mesothelioma	Olaparib	2	NCT03531840

Study title	Drug interventions	Phase	NCT number
Anti-Mesothelin Immunotoxin LMB-100 Followed by Pembrolizumab in Malignant Mesothelioma	LMB-100, Pembrolizumab	2	NCT03644550

**Completed.*
***Suspended/terminated.*

Table 1.
Highlighted drug-based clinical trials for mesothelioma from clinicaltrials.gov (U.S. National Library of Medicine).

and pemetrexed as a first-line treatment for unresectable pleural mesothelioma has also been reported to be advancing to a larger randomized phase III trial [5, 39]. Pembrolizumab is a PD-1 (which binds to PD-L1) inhibitor currently being used for a phase II/III trial (NCT02784171) for advanced pleural mesothelioma both as a monotherapy (phase II) and in combination with cisplatin and pemetrexed (phase III). Nivolumab is a PD-1 inhibitor in two phase III clinical trials, which are for relapsed mesothelioma (NCT03063450) and as a first-line treatment when combined with ipilimumab for unresectable pleural mesothelioma (NCT02899299). Ipilimumab is a cytotoxic T-lymphocyte-associated protein 4 (CTLA-4) inhibitor that has showed encouraging results when previously combined with nivolumab in two separate phase II trials for mesothelioma [40, 41]. The CTLA-4 inhibitor tremelimumab was reported to be unsuccessful as a second-line treatment in two phase II clinical trials. As a monotherapy, it did not prolong overall survival for both unresectable pleural and peritoneal mesothelioma (NCT01843374) [42] and the primary endpoint for overall response rate was not met when tested in combination with durvalumab for pleural mesothelioma (NCT03075527) [43].

The PD-1 inhibitor pembrolizumab is also being combined with the focal adhesion kinase inhibitor defactinib in a phase 1 clinical trial (NCT04201145). There had previously been a lot of interest in the ability of focal adhesion kinase inhibition to selectively eliminate mesothelioma cells, but enthusiasm significantly decreased after defactinib failed to improve progression-free and overall survival in prior mesothelioma clinical trials (NCT02004028, NCT01870609) [44]. However, defactinib is now also in the MATCH screening phase II trial for patients with advanced refractory solid tumors containing *NF2* inactivating mutations as a second-line treatment (NCT02465060, subprotocol U). This is the only current clinical trial (to the best of our knowledge) that may potentially address inactivating *NF2* mutations in mesothelioma (note that the trial is not specific to mesothelioma and does not guarantee mesothelioma patient enrollment). The mTOR inhibitor everolimus had been previously studied in a second-line mesothelioma phase II trial that also evaluated NF2 loss as a biomarker of sensitivity (NCT01024946), but this trial resulted in limited clinical activity and everolimus did not progress as a monotherapy agent for mesothelioma [45]. In preclinical studies, we have found that repurposing the antimalarial drug quinacrine may be particularly effective against cells with inactivating *NF2* mutations by disrupting hippo signaling (*unpublished data*). Quinacrine is unique as an anticancer agent in that it has an excellent safety profile from almost a century of use for malaria prophylaxis/treatment [46]. Further mechanistic and clinical studies are needed to fully understand the potential of quinacrine for mesothelioma treatment. Moreover, verteporfin has also been preclinically evaluated as a YAP inhibitor for mesothelioma, but has not progressed to clinical trials yet [29, 30]. To address BAP1 inactivation, a phase II trial testing the EZH2 inhibitor tazemetostat with relapsed/refractory mesothelioma patients as a monotherapy (NCT02860286) recently concluded with encouraging preliminary data, specifically benefiting long-term disease control [47]. Targeting *BAP1*-mutated mesothelioma tumors with poly-ADP-ribose-polymerase (PARP) inhibitors has been promising based on preclinical studies [48, 49]. The PARP inhibitor niraparib is being evaluated as a second-line treatment in a phase II trial for tumors with DNA damage response mutations including *BAP1* (NCT03207347). More recently, a phase II trial to evaluate the PARP inhibitor olaparib as a second-line treatment specifically for mesothelioma has started with arms to include *BAP1* somatic mutations and germline DNA damage repair mutations (NCT03531840). The MiST phase II trial also has an arm for investigating the PARP inhibitor rucaparib in BRCA1/BAP1-negative mesothelioma patients. Furthermore, the MiST trial has a third arm to study the CDK4/6 inhibitor abemaciclib for mesothelioma patients with p16INK4A negative (*CDKN2A* deletion) tumors. The fourth MiST arm evaluates AXL inhibitor bemcentinib in combination with pembrolizumab for relapsed mesothelioma patients without specific biomarker requirements. We have previously shown that AXL has relatively high expression in pleural mesothelioma compared to other cancer types, and that bemcentinib can selectively kill mesothelioma cells [50]. In pleural mesothelioma, a phase II trial with epidermal growth factor receptor (EGFR) inhibitor gefitinib was not successful [51]. However, peritoneal mesothelioma often has higher EGFR expression compared to pleural mesothelioma and may benefit from EGFR inhibitor therapy pending more clinical studies that are specific for this indication [2, 52].

Mesothelin and other biomarkers of mesothelioma have gained recent interest as targets for immunotoxins and chimeric antigen receptor-T (CAR-T) cells. Mesothelin has been used for diagnostic purposes in algorithms with other biomarkers as well as occasionally used for tumor surveillance [2, 5]. As a therapy target, the immunotoxin LMB-100 has been recently developed to bind mesothelin [53]. In 2018, a phase II trial started with LMB-100 followed by pembrolizumab for pleural and peritoneal mesothelioma cohorts (NCT03644550). CAR-T cells are also being developed to target mesothelin as a potential mesothelioma treatment [54].

5. Conclusions

Most mesothelioma patients have chemotherapy or experimental drugs as a major part of their treatment plan, but there have been very few highlights and minimal significant advancements for mesothelioma drugs over the last couple decades. Targeting specific types and characteristics of mesothelioma may have the most potential in the near future. It is surprising that targeted drugs as a whole have not progressed to end stages already either because of slower development pipelines or failure to hit endpoints for mesothelioma. There may also be an orphan drug clout that prevents development of drugs to target tumors with *BAP1* and *NF2* mutations. Proteomic characteristics of mesothelioma, specifically biomarkers currently used for diagnostic and tumor surveillance purposes, may also prove useful for novel chimeric therapies (e.g. protac and chimeric antigen receptor T cells), which are currently being developed for mesothelin. These and emerging targeted drugs such as AXL inhibitors, EGFR inhibitors for peritoneal mesothelioma, PARP inhibitors for *BAP1*-mutated tumors, and quinacrine for *NF2*-mutated tumors all have potential to finally kill the reputation of mesothelioma as a drug development graveyard.

Acknowledgements

This work was supported in part by grants from the Department of Laboratory Medicine and Pathology at the Mayo Clinic (Molina and Shridhar) and the

American Cancer Society—Kirby Foundation Postdoctoral Fellowship (Oien, PF-17-241-01-CCG). These sponsors had no involvement in any of the design or writing of this article. The authors thank Caleb Swalve for assistance in preparing this manuscript.

Conflict of interest

The authors have no conflicts of interest to declare.

Author details

Derek B. Oien[1], Jeremy Chien[2], Julian Molina[1] and Viji Shridhar[1]*

1 Mayo Clinic, Rochester, Minnesota, USA

2 University of California Davis Health, Sacramento, California, USA

*Address all correspondence to: shridhar.vijayalakshmi@mayo.edu

References

[1] Henley SJ, Larson TC, Wu M, Antao VC, Lewis M, Pinheiro GA, et al. Mesothelioma incidence in 50 states and the District of Columbia, United States, 2003-2008. International Journal of Occupational and Environmental Health. 2013;**19**:1-10

[2] Kim J, Bhagwandin S, Labow DM. Malignant peritoneal mesothelioma: A review. Annals of Translational Medicine. 2017;**5**:236

[3] Brenner J, Sordillo PP, Magill GB, Golbey RB. Malignant mesothelioma of the pleura: Review of 123 patients. Cancer. 1982;**49**:2431-2435

[4] Finn RS, Brims FJH, Gandhi A, Olsen N, Musk AW, Maskell NA, et al. Postmortem findings of malignant pleural mesothelioma: A two-center study of 318 patients. Chest. 2012;**142**:1267-1273

[5] Carbone M, Adusumilli PS, Alexander HR Jr, Baas P, Bardelli F, Bononi A, et al. Mesothelioma: Scientific clues for prevention, diagnosis, and therapy. CA: A Cancer Journal for Clinicians. 2019;**69**:402-429

[6] Sugarbaker PH. Update on the management of malignant peritoneal mesothelioma. Translational Lung Cancer Research. 2018;**7**:599-608

[7] Vogelzang NJ, Rusthoven JJ, Symanowski J, Denham C, Kaukel E, Ruffie P, et al. Phase III study of pemetrexed in combination with cisplatin versus cisplatin alone in patients with malignant pleural mesothelioma. Journal of Clinical Oncology: Official Journal of the American Society of Clinical Oncology. 2003;**21**:2636-2644

[8] Campbell NP, Kindler HL. Update on malignant pleural mesothelioma. Seminars in Respiratory and Critical Care Medicine. 2011;**32**:102-110

[9] Simon GR, Verschraegen CF, Janne PA, Langer CJ, Dowlati A, Gadgeel SM, et al. Pemetrexed plus gemcitabine as first-line chemotherapy for patients with peritoneal mesothelioma: Final report of a phase II trial. Journal of Clinical Oncology: Official Journal of the American Society of Clinical Oncology. 2008;**26**:3567-3572

[10] Le DT, Deavers M, Hunt K, Malpica A, Verschraegen CF. Cisplatin and irinotecan (CPT-11) for peritoneal mesothelioma. Cancer Investigation. 2003;**21**:682-689

[11] Steele JP, Shamash J, Evans MT, Gower NH, Tischkowitz MD, Rudd RM. Phase II study of vinorelbine in patients with malignant pleural mesothelioma. Journal of Clinical Oncology: Official Journal of the American Society of Clinical Oncology. 2000;**18**:3912-3917

[12] Yan TD, Deraco M, Baratti D, Kusamura S, Elias D, Glehen O, et al. Cytoreductive surgery and hyperthermic intraperitoneal chemotherapy for malignant peritoneal mesothelioma: Multi-institutional experience. Journal of Clinical Oncology: Official Journal of the American Society of Clinical Oncology. 2009;**27**:6237-6242

[13] Alexander HR Jr, Bartlett DL, Pingpank JF, Libutti SK, Royal R, Hughes MS, et al. Treatment factors associated with long-term survival after cytoreductive surgery and regional chemotherapy for patients with malignant peritoneal mesothelioma. Surgery. 2013;**153**:779-786

[14] Pretorius RG, Petrilli ES, Kean CK, Ford LC, Hoeschele JD, Lagasse LD. Comparison of the iv and

ip routes of administration of cisplatin in dogs. Cancer Treatment Reports. 1981;**65**:1055-1062

[15] Neuwirth MG, Alexander HR, Karakousis GC. Then and now: Cytoreductive surgery with hyperthermic intraperitoneal chemotherapy (HIPEC), a historical perspective. Journal of Gastrointestinal Oncology. 2016;**7**:18-28

[16] Dedrick RL, Myers CE, Bungay PM, DeVita VT Jr. Pharmacokinetic rationale for peritoneal drug administration in the treatment of ovarian cancer. Cancer Treatment Reports. 1978;**62**:1-11

[17] Bueno R, Stawiski EW, Goldstein LD, Durinck S, De Rienzo A, Modrusan Z, et al. Comprehensive genomic analysis of malignant pleural mesothelioma identifies recurrent mutations, gene fusions and splicing alterations. Nature Genetics. 2016;**48**:407-416

[18] Hmeljak J, Sanchez-Vega F, Hoadley KA. Integrative molecular characterization of malignant pleural mesothelioma. Cancer Discovery. 2018;**8**:1548-1565

[19] Al Sarakbi W, Sasi W, Jiang WG, Roberts T, Newbold RF, Mokbel K. The mRNA expression of SETD2 in human breast cancer: Correlation with clinico-pathological parameters. BMC Cancer. 2009;**9**:290

[20] Testa JR, Cheung M, Pei J, Below JE, Tan Y, Sementino E, et al. Germline BAP1 mutations predispose to malignant mesothelioma. Nature Genetics. 2011;**43**:1022-1025

[21] Guo G, Chmielecki J, Goparaju C, Heguy A, Dolgalev I, Carbone M, et al. Whole-exome sequencing reveals frequent genetic alterations in BAP1, NF2, CDKN2A, and CUL1 in malignant pleural mesothelioma. Cancer Research. 2015;**75**:264-269

[22] Nasu M, Emi M, Pastorino S, Tanji M, Powers A, Luk H, et al. High incidence of somatic BAP1 alterations in sporadic malignant mesothelioma. Journal of Thoracic Oncology: Official Publication of the International Association for the Study of Lung Cancer. 2015;**10**:565-576

[23] Yoshikawa Y, Emi M, Hashimoto-Tamaoki T, Ohmuraya M, Sato A, Tsujimura T, et al. High-density array-CGH with targeted NGS unmask multiple noncontiguous minute deletions on chromosome 3p21 in mesothelioma. Proceedings of the National Academy of Sciences of the United States of America. 2016;**113**:13432-13437

[24] Bononi A, Giorgi C, Patergnani S, Larson D, Verbruggen K, Tanji M, et al. BAP1 regulates IP3R3-mediated Ca^{2+} flux to mitochondria suppressing cell transformation. Nature. 2017;**546**:549-553

[25] Bononi A, Yang H, Giorgi C, Patergnani S, Pellegrini L, Su M, et al. Germline BAP1 mutations induce a Warburg effect. Cell Death & Differentiation. 2017;**24**:1694-1704

[26] LaFave LM, Beguelin W, Koche R, Teater M, Spitzer B, Chramiec A, et al. Loss of BAP1 function leads to EZH2-dependent. Transformation. 2015;**21**:1344-1349

[27] Walpole S, Pritchard AL, Cebulla CM, Pilarski R, Stautberg M, Davidorf FH, et al. Comprehensive study of the clinical phenotype of germline BAP1 variant-carrying families worldwide. Journal of the National Cancer Institute. 2018;**110**:1328-1341

[28] Petrilli AM, Fernandez-Valle C. Role of Merlin/NF2 inactivation in tumor biology. Oncogene. 2016;**35**:537-548

[29] Zhang WQ, Dai YY. Targeting YAP in malignant pleural mesothelioma.

Journal of Cellular and Molecular Medicine. 2017;**21**:2663-2676

[30] Tranchant R, Quetel L, Tallet A, Meiller C, Renier A, de Koning L, et al. Co-occurring mutations of tumor suppressor genes, LATS2 and NF2, in malignant pleural mesothelioma. Clinical Cancer Research: An Official Journal of the American Association for Cancer Research. 2017;**23**:3191-3202

[31] Sekido Y, Pass HI, Bader S, Mew DJ, Christman MF, Gazdar AF, et al. Neurofibromatosis type 2 (NF2) gene is somatically mutated in mesothelioma but not in lung cancer. Cancer Research. 1995;**55**:1227-1231

[32] Bianchi AB, Mitsunaga SI, Cheng JQ, Klein WM, Jhanwar SC, Seizinger B, et al. High frequency of inactivating mutations in the neurofibromatosis type 2 gene (NF2) in primary malignant mesotheliomas. Proceedings of the National Academy of Sciences of the United States of America. 1995;**92**:10854-10858

[33] Mansfield AS, Peikert T, Smadbeck JB, Udell JBM, Garcia-Rivera E, Elsbernd L, et al. Neoantigenic potential of complex chromosomal rearrangements in mesothelioma. Journal of Thoracic Oncology: Official Publication of the International Association for the Study of Lung Cancer. 2019;**14**:276-287

[34] Zalcman G, Mazieres J, Margery J, Greillier L, Audigier-Valette C, Moro-Sibilot D, et al. Bevacizumab for newly diagnosed pleural mesothelioma in the mesothelioma Avastin Cisplatin Pemetrexed study (MAPS): A randomised, controlled, open-label, phase 3 trial. Lancet (London, England). 2016;**387**:1405-1414

[35] Eberst G, Anota A, Scherpereel A, Mazieres J. Health-related quality of life impact from adding bevacizumab to cisplatin-pemetrexed in malignant pleural mesothelioma in the MAPS IFCT-GFPC-0701 phase III trial. Clinical Cancer Research. 2019;**25**:5759-5765

[36] Tsao AS, Miao J, Wistuba II, Vogelzang NJ, Heymach JV, Fossella FV, et al. Phase II trial of cediranib in combination with cisplatin and pemetrexed in chemotherapy-naive patients with unresectable malignant pleural mesothelioma (SWOG S0905). Journal of Clinical Oncology: Official Journal of the American Society of Clinical Oncology. 2019;**37**:2537-2547

[37] Buikhuisen WA, Scharpfenecker M, Griffioen AW, Korse CM, van Tinteren H, Baas P, et al. Study adding axitinib to pemetrexed-cisplatin in patients with malignant pleural mesothelioma: A single-center trial combining clinical and translational outcomes. Journal of Thoracic Oncology: Official Publication of the International Association for the Study of Lung Cancer. 2016;**11**:758-768

[38] Scagliotti GV, Gaafar R, Nowak AK, Nakano T, van Meerbeeck J, Popat S, et al. Nintedanib in combination with pemetrexed and cisplatin for chemotherapy-naive patients with advanced malignant pleural mesothelioma (LUME-Meso): A double-blind, randomised, placebo-controlled phase 3 trial. The Lancer Respiratory Medicine. 2019;**7**:569-580

[39] Nowak A, Kok P, Lesterhuis W, Hughes B, Brown C, Kao S, et al. OA08.02 DREAM-A phase 2 trial of durvalumab with first line chemotherapy in mesothelioma: Final result. Journal of Thoracic Oncology. 2018;**13**:S338-S339

[40] Disselhorst MJ, Quispel-Janssen J, Lalezari F, Monkhorst K, de Vries JF, van der Noort V, et al. Ipilimumab and nivolumab in the treatment of recurrent malignant pleural mesothelioma (INITIATE): Results of a prospective,

single-arm, phase 2 trial. The Lancet Respiratory Medicine. 2019;7:260-270

[41] Scherpereel A, Mazieres J, Greillier L, Lantuejoul S, Do P, Bylicki O, et al. Nivolumab or nivolumab plus ipilimumab in patients with relapsed malignant pleural mesothelioma (IFCT-1501 MAPS2): A multicentre, open-label, randomised, non-comparative, phase 2 trial. The Lancet. Oncology. 2019;**20**:239-253

[42] Maio M, Scherpereel A, Calabro L, Aerts J, Cedres Perez S, Bearz A, et al. Tremelimumab as second-line or third-line treatment in relapsed malignant mesothelioma (DETERMINE): A multicentre, international, randomised, double-blind, placebo-controlled phase 2b trial. The Lancet. Oncology. 2017;**18**:1261-1273

[43] Venkatraman D, Anderson A, Digumarthy S, Lizotte PH, Awad MM. Phase 2 study of tremelimumab plus durvalumab for previously-treated malignant pleural mesothelioma (MPM). Journal of Clinical Oncology. 2019;**37**:8549-8549

[44] Fennell DA, Baas P, Taylor P, Nowak AK, Gilligan D, Nakano T, et al. Maintenance defactinib versus placebo after first-line chemotherapy in patients with merlin-stratified pleural mesothelioma: COMMAND-A double-blind, randomized, Phase II study. Journal of Clinical Oncology: Official Journal of the American Society of Clinical Oncology. 2019;**37**:790-798

[45] Ou SH, Moon J, Garland LL, Mack PC, Testa JR, Tsao AS, et al. SWOG S0722: Phase II study of mTOR inhibitor everolimus (RAD001) in advanced malignant pleural mesothelioma (MPM). Journal of Thoracic Oncology: Official Publication of the International Association for the Study of Lung Cancer. 2015;**10**:387-391

[46] Oien DB, Pathoulas CL, Ray U, Thirusangu P, Kalogera E, Shridhar V. Repurposing quinacrine for treatment-refractory cancer. Seminars in Cancer Biology. 2019

[47] Zauderer MG, Szlosarek P, Moulec SL, Popat S, Taylor P, Planchard D, et al. Phase 2, multicenter study of the EZH2 inhibitor tazemetostat as monotherapy in adults with relapsed or refractory (R/R) malignant mesothelioma (MM) with BAP1 inactivation. Journal of Clinical Oncology. 2018;**36**:8515-8515

[48] Borchert S, Wessolly M, Schmeller J, Mairinger E, Kollmeier J, Hager T, et al. Gene expression profiling of homologous recombination repair pathway indicates susceptibility for olaparib treatment in malignant pleural mesothelioma in vitro. BMC Cancer. 2019;**19**:108

[49] Parrotta R, Okonska A, Ronner M, Weder W, Stahel R, Penengo L, et al. A novel BRCA1-associated protein-1 isoform affects response of mesothelioma cells to drugs impairing BRCA1-mediated DNA repair. Journal of Thoracic Oncology: Official Publication of the International Association for the Study of Lung Cancer. 2017;**12**:1309-1319

[50] Oien DB, Garay T, Eckstein S, Chien J. Cisplatin and pemetrexed activate AXL and AXL inhibitor BGB324 enhances mesothelioma cell death from chemotherapy. Frontiers in Pharmacology. 2017;**8**:970

[51] Govindan R, Kratzke RA, Herndon JE 2nd, Niehans GA, Vollmer R, Watson D, et al. Gefitinib in patients with malignant mesothelioma: A phase II study by the cancer and leukemia group B. Clinical Cancer Research: An Official Journal of the American Association for Cancer Research. 2005;**11**:2300-2304

[52] Foster JM, Radhakrishna U, Govindarajan V, Carreau JH, Gatalica Z, Sharma P, et al. Clinical implications of novel activating EGFR mutations in malignant peritoneal mesothelioma. World Journal of Surgical Oncology. 2010;**8**:88

[53] Zhang J, Khanna S, Jiang Q, Alewine C, Miettinen M, Pastan I, et al. Efficacy of anti-mesothelin Immunotoxin RG7787 plus nab-paclitaxel against mesothelioma patient-derived xenografts and mesothelin as a biomarker of tumor response. Clinical Cancer Research: An Official Journal of the American Association for Cancer Research. 2017;**23**:1564-1574

[54] Ye L, Lou Y, Lu L, Fan X. Mesothelin-targeted second generation CAR-T cells inhibit growth of mesothelin-expressing tumors in vivo. Experimental and Therapeutic Medicine. 2019;**17**:739-747

Section 4

Predictive and Prognostic Biomarkers

Chapter 5

Predictive and Prognosis Factors of Clinical Utility in Mesothelioma

Rodríguez-Cid Jeronimo Rafael
and Flores-Mariñelarena Rodrigo Rafael

Abstract

The constant research in therapeutics for mesothelioma has been improving their tumor response and overall survival, generating the need to propose markers that guide the doctor's therapeutic approach in a more precise way. Recently, different predictive factors have been proposed, such as mesothelin-related peptides, fibulin-3, and osteopontin associated with an image giving information about the probability of tumor response to a therapeutic agent or a combination of agents. As is well known, the importance of prognostic markers of utility lies in providing prospective information on the evolution of the patient and thus their ability to guide therapeutic decisions. Although the clinical stage and histology are currently the most described prognostic factors, recent studies have shown interest in the expression of estrogen receptor beta and calretinin, among other promising factors. Given the heterogeneity of this broad field of research in mesothelioma, it is necessary to objectively present the prognostic and predictive factors of greater clinical utility.

Keywords: prognosis factors, predictive factors, response to treatment, clinical factors, histopathology factors, biological factors, clinical scores

1. Introduction

The prognosis of patients with mesothelioma is unfavorable, with a median survival of approximately 12 months from diagnosis [1–5]; this makes a clear need to improve the effectiveness of multimodality approaches and to define in a better way the subgroups' prognosis [6–9]. One way to achieve this objective is the use of prognostic and predictive factors; a prognostic factor provides prospective information on the evolution of the patient being able to guide therapeutic decisions, while a predictive factor gives us information on the probability of tumor response to a therapeutic agent.

The characteristics that a prognostic factor must meet are: (a) simple prediction method, (b) wide availability, (c) sensitivity, and (d) reproducibility in any clinical situation. The purpose of these markers is to help define the individual prognosis of clinical groups, select patients who may need other treatments, and assign the most effective treatments to improve survival and quality of life.

Although currently the therapeutic decisions are still based on the classic clinical and pathological prognostic factors already known, such as age, functional status, sex, chest pain, weight loss, thrombocytosis, leukocytosis, anemia, and histological type [3, 10], biological and genetic factors may soon be excellent options as prognostic and predictive factors.

2. Clinical factors

Multiple mesothelioma series have validated advanced TNM stage, age $\geq$ 50 years, male gender, poor performance status, weight loss, platelet counts $\geq$400,000, white blood cell counts $\geq$15.5, low hemoglobin level, low albumin levels, and high serum lactate dehydrogenase levels, among others, as poor predictive and prognosis factors [11–21].

TNM stage is one of the most studied prognosis factors describing a poor survival prognosis for those with advanced or metastatic stage, however, in the same stage of the disease, patients' survival varies widely suggesting that TNM staging is not completely precise to predict a survival outcome [16]. Moreover, with the new changes applied since the release of the eighth edition of the TNM Classification for Lung and Pleural Tumors where all patients N0M0 malignant pleural mesothelioma as stage IA or IB, differing from the seventh edition classification, in which N0 also was listed within the classifications for stages II and III. These changes reclassified as stage I many patients who were formerly considered as stage II or III since some patients at stage IB experienced poorer prognosis than those at stage III [22, 23]. Identifying prognostic factors based on the new classification should help to identify the patients with a poor prognosis who may benefit from multimodality treatments. Additional to the TNM staging system, the true tumor volume was independently associated with overall survival and response to treatment; however, more studies need to be done to validate this variable [24–27].

Previous studies have suggested that females with mesothelioma experience longer survival compared to males [6, 28–33] with possible suggested explications like those they present at earlier stage [34], tumors with more favorable histology [30], different asbestos exposure responsible for a more indolent tumor biology [35], and a protective effect of circulating estrogen interacting with estrogen receptors present in their tumors, [32, 36, 37] however, only more indolent tumor biology associated to higher frequency of germline mutations in DNA repair genes [38–41] and interaction of estrogens with estrogen receptor beta [36, 37, 42, 43], other theories still controversial [15].

Platelet count is a practical and easy blood test in clinical practice that has been studied for its role as a prognosis factor due to the interaction of platelets with tumor cells contributing to tumor progression, invasion, metastasis, and angiogenesis [44]. This interaction could be explained by five possible pathways: the first one refers to the release of growth factor by the platelets, including transforming growth factor β and fibroblast growth factor enhancing cancer cell proliferation [45]. Second, platelet membranes are rich in many adhesin molecules like selectins, integrins, immunoglobulin superfamily proteins, and leucine-rich glycoproteins stabilizing the cancer cell arrest in the vasculature, increasing potential of metastasis [46]. Third, platelets could mediate the invasive potential of cancer cells by the release of thromboxane A2, 12-hydroxyeicosatetranoic acid, and matrix metalloproteinases [47–49]. Fourth, platelets release a large number of pro-angiogenic mediators such as vascular endothelial growth factor and basic fibroblast growth factor influencing the tumor angiogenesis and consequently tumor growth [50–52]. Fifth, some studies have demonstrated that platelets facilitate the immune escape of cancer cells by surrounding tumor cells and protecting them from the cytotoxic effect of natural killer cells [53, 54]. Several studies concluded that thrombocytosis is correlated with worse overall survival in patients with mesothelioma, indicating that pretreatment could be an adequate and useful factor of prognosis [18].

Recently, many people have focused on the role of inflammation in cancer due to its contribution to tumor initiation and malignant progression. More specifically in mesothelioma, inflammation becomes relevant since most patients have a history of asbestos exposure, and this mineral can skewer cells and set off chemical reactions that lead to inflammation, DNA damage, and cell death [20]. Leukocyte blood count reflects a degree of the systemic inflammatory response in tumor patients, being a valuable and simple indicator [55]. Blood neutrophil-to-lymphocyte ratio is a systemic marker for inflammation closely related to the mortality rate and response to the treatment is useful as a predictive and prognostic factor, taking 3 as a dividing point [20, 56–60]. In the same way, serum c-protein can reflect an inflammatory environment; although its usefulness as a prognostic and predictive factor has been demonstrated in limited studies, more research is needed to validate its utility [61–63].

Malnutrition has been related to adverse outcomes in overall survival, quality of life, and increased mortality of malignant tumors [64–66]. Serum albumin level is a simple and objective indicator to evaluate malnutrition. Multiple studies have demonstrated hypoalbuminemia as an adverse independent prognostic factor for mesothelioma [19, 20, 67].

It is well known that cancer cells tend to employ alternate metabolic pathways, generating adenosine triphosphate through anaerobic glycolysis regulated by lactate dehydrogenase [68, 69]. Several studies assessed the value of high pretreatment lactate dehydrogenase levels for the prediction of a worse survival outcome in mesothelioma [10, 61, 62, 70–75]. The association between high lactate dehydrogenase levels and poor prognosis on malignancies has tried to be explained in multiple ways. The first theory implies that the production of lactate acid could be up-regulated by lactate dehydrogenase, generating an acidic environment activating metalloproteases, macrophage-mediated angiogenesis and protecting mitochondria from oxidative stress, which induces resistance to hypoxia-induced apoptosis of tumor cells [76–80]. The second theory explains a strong correlation between elevated lactate dehydrogenase levels and an up-regulation of the hypoxia-inducible factor pathway resulting in a host immunological function attenuation, and enhanced tumor angiogenesis, which has an adverse impact on prognosis in malignant tumors [81]. Despite the great evidence of the utility of lactate dehydrogenase as a convenient and cost-effective indicator for predicting overall survival outcome, cut-off values of lactate dehydrogenase reported on the literature are inconsistent, and it is important to standardize the cut-off value in future studies.

3. Histopathology factors

Together with the TNM stage, the histological type is one of the strongest prognostic factors among patients with mesothelioma. However, with the support of immunohistochemistry markers, not only has diagnosis been improved, but also new markers have appeared for a more accurate prediction of response to treatment, overall survival, and developing better therapeutic approaches.

The most significant prognostic factor until now remains histology with a better prognosis for epithelioid type than sarcomatoid or biphasic type mesothelioma [10, 12, 82, 83]. In addition to histologic subtyping (with solid growth pattern being associated with a poor outcome), nuclear atypia, mitotic count, and the presence of necrosis were found to be independent prognostic factors in epithelioid malignant pleural mesothelioma [84–86].

Ki67 antigen is used for the assessment of growth fraction of cell populations, due to it being exclusively expressed in proliferating cells; cell cycle analysis showed that Ki67 is detectable in G1, G2, S, and mitosis phases but absent in quiescent cells [87, 88]. Despite most studies indicating that high expression of Ki67 leads to a poor prognosis, some malignancies showing high Ki67 levels actually show a better response to treatment, which could be explained by the fact that cells with high proliferation are susceptible to cytotoxic agents [89–93]. The detection of Ki67 is not a routine procedure for mesothelioma's diagnosis and treatment; however, a group has suggested to consider it due to its utility as a possible prognostic marker in epithelioid mesothelioma with a better prognosis outcome in those with low expression levels [94–98].

Calretinin is a calcium-binding protein that has been established as a useful marker in distinguishing mesothelioma from adenocarcinomas with pleural metastases [99]; Additionally, interest in using higher calretinin scores as favorable prognostic factors has been growing, although further investigation is needed [100–104].

As mentioned above in the section of clinical factors, estrogen receptor beta expressed on mesothelial tumor cells has become a promising prognostic factor and a possible future therapeutic target [36, 37, 42, 43].

4. Biological factors

Several biomarkers are selectively elevated in patients with mesothelioma. However, further study and validation are required before they are recommended as routine predictive or prognosis factors and they should be adjunct to a radiological assessment. With considerable variation in response to treatment, the emergence of promising biomarkers that could select responders from non-responders at baseline or during treatment would guide to a better therapeutic approach, prevent patients from getting ineffective treatments, and improve cost-effectiveness.

The most researched biomarker until now is the mesothelin; soluble mesothelin is a circulating form of a membrane-bound glycoprotein highly expressed by mesothelial cells in mesothelioma (predominantly epithelioid type) and other malignancies [105]. Despite the controversial evidence reported in the literature [106–114], a meta-analysis conducted by Tian et al. [115] concluded that a high soluble mesothelin level may lead to a poor prognosis for patients with mesothelioma, it being appropriate to consider mesothelin level as an independent prognostic marker.

Human fibulin-3 is a secreted glycoprotein that plays an essential role in the regulation of cell proliferation and migration [116, 117]. Recent findings have documented altered levels on patients with mesothelioma, highlighting them as a novel biomarker for this malignancy; however, as most studies have been done with limited sample size [114, 118–120], and the results may not completely mirror the actual value of fibulin-3 for prognosis, further studies are needed for a more comprehensive prognostic role of human fibulin-3 in mesothelioma.

Osteopontin is a glycoprotein that mediates cell-matrix interactions with adverse outcomes for mesothelioma [98, 121, 122]; however, its utility is limited because of the significant variability in the cut-offs used between studies. In order to be validated in the future, a consensus approach is required for sampling and analysis [122].

CA 125 is a transmembrane glycoprotein that can be detected in the fallopian tube, endometrium, endocervix, and mesothelial surface of the peritoneum, pleura, and pericardium [98]. Some cases with non-gynecological cancer showed positive immunohistochemical staining for CA125 in tumor tissue and elevated CA 125 levels in serum [123–125]. The baseline levels of serum CA125 accompanied by the stage of the disease could be used as independent prognostic factors for patients with mesothelioma; the change in serum CA125 levels can predict overall survival and response to systemic treatments [126–128].

5. Clinical scores

The best-known clinical prognostic scoring systems for mesothelioma until now derive from the Cancer and Leukemia Group B (CALGB) and the European

Organization for Research and Treatment of Cancer (EORTC), both scores have been widely used to better select patients who have a favorable prognosis and could tolerate and potentially benefit from a more aggressive combined modality treatment [3, 10].

The CALGB index was validated by examining the survival of a wide cohort dividing patients into six patient subgroups with different survival rates. The CALGB study considered extent pleural disease, lactate dehydrogenase >500 UI/L, poor performance status, platelets >400,000, non-epithelial histology, and >75 years as negative prognostic factors for survival. The most favorable characteristics were a performance status of 0, age < 49, and hemoglobin ≥14.6/μl [10].

The EORTC score has been validated in 523 patients included in 10 mesothelioma trials with the analysis suggesting that performance status >0, stage IV disease, and biphasic or sarcomatous histologies are associated with a worse outcome [129]. Additional reports confirmed that male sex, older age, and abnormal hematological values also give a poor prognosis [13, 130].

Despite both studies identifying performance status and histology as two main prognostic factors, these analyses included patients with heterogeneous tumor stages at diagnosis, the majority of whom underwent major surgery and whose treatment predated the use of pemetrexed as first-line treatment. Since the positioning of pemetrexed as a first-line treatment, no validated prognostic score has appeared, resulting in the need to generate new studies with the aforementioned scores [131].

6. Promising factors

Although there are multiple prognostic and predictive factors that are currently validated, many others have generated great interest for their potential as a therapeutic target in the future.

There is an increasing interest in the use of semi-quantitative ^{18}F-FDG PET/CT parameters, like metabolic tumor volume and total lesion glycolysis to measure the metabolic activity in the entire tumor volume with great potential to predict response to treatment [119, 132–144]; however further investigation is needed in mesothelioma patients.

Despite the wide utility of the tissue biopsy, the invasive nature limits their application, especially when repeated biopsies are needed. Given the aforementioned, liquid biopsy has gained interest from oncologists and basic researchers [145]. Although liquid biopsy is still far from replacing tissue biopsy for mesothelioma, plasma and serum samples represent minimally invasive, low-risk, and easily obtained biological fluids that many studies have indicated as potentially interesting prognosis biomarkers as mentioned in the section "Biological factors" [146].

Nowadays, immunotherapy is gaining great relevance in cancer therapeutics. Soon, oncologists will routinely ask for programmed death-ligand 1 (PD-L1) status that has been correlated with better treatment response to anti-PD-L1 antibodies and overall survival outcomes [147–151]. However, different PD-L1 antibodies coupled with specific staining platforms and scoring criteria may be necessary since finding a suitable cut-off point remains a current challenge [151, 152].

A wide number of molecular prognostic markers for mesothelioma have been investigated. The number of tumor-infiltrating myeloid cells, c-MET expression, thymidylate synthase expression, among others, represent promising biomarkers associated with strong prognostic significance. c-MET is a tyrosine kinase receptor, its overexpression was associated with longer overall survival in patients with mesothelioma [98, 153]. Thymidylate synthase expression may predict pemetrexed efficacy, a certain correlation has also been found with overall survival and progression-free survival [154].

Dysregulated genes play a critical role in the development and progression of mesothelioma, making them future diagnosis and prognosis biomarkers [155]. Recently, Zhou et al. obtained an RNA-Seq count quantified by RSEM for RNA expression profiles of a large cohort of patients with mesothelioma according to The Cancer Genome Atlas guidelines. After a time-dependent receiver operated a characteristic curve to evaluate the prognostic performance of survival prediction, three genes (LSM6, GZMB, and HJURP) were found with a strong statistically significant prognostic association; this prognostic signature could be a clinically useful tool that in the future could be incorporated into a clinical sequencing program to individualize therapy [156].

7. Conclusion

Despite the wide variety of predictive and prognostic factors that exist, just a few are replicable worldwide. Furthermore, only pathological type and performance status are the grade-A recommendations of prognostic factors in pretreatment assessment, as well as the nodal stage, residual disease, and histology during treatment [16].

Although there is currently no validated prognostic approach, according to individual evidence, availability, and cost-benefit, it is recommended to pay special attention to the TNM classification, histological type, and serum CA125 in the decision for multimodal therapy. Despite the practicality of the prognostic scoring systems, further investigations are needed to validate the known scores or generated new ones that fit the new existing therapeutic modalities for mesothelioma.

In the near future, many other prognostic and predictive factors may be introduced in clinical practice making a selection of mesothelioma subgroups to improve the benefit achievable by currently available treatment strategies, and relentless efforts will have to be focused on designing innovative compounds selectively targeting the existing (or additional) markers to improve the grim prognosis of the disease.

Conflict of interest

Dr. Jeronimo Rafael Rodríguez-Cid has educational, investigational and advice relations with MSD, Bristol Myers, Roche, Takeda, Amgen, Abvie, Aztra Zeneca, Boehringer Ingelheim, Pfizer, Celgen, Novartis, and Bayer.

Dr. Rodrigo Rafael Flores-Mariñelarena have no conflicts of interest to declare.

Notes/Thanks/Other declarations

None to declare.

Author details

Rodríguez-Cid Jeronimo Rafael[1]* and Flores-Mariñelarena Rodrigo Rafael[2]

1 Department of Oncology, Instituto Nacional de Enfermedades Respiratorias Ismael Cosío Villegas, Mexico City, Mexico

2 Department of Internal Medicine, Fundación Clínica Médica Sur, Mexico City, Mexico

*Address all correspondence to: cidjeronimo@yahoo.com.mx

References

[1] Ruffe PA. Pleural mesothelioma. Current Opinion in Oncology. 1991;**3**(2):328-334

[2] de Pangher MV, Brollo A, Franceschi S, de Matthaeis M, Talamini R, Bianchi C. Prognostic factors of malignant mesothelioma of the pleura. Cancer. 1993;**72**(2):410-417

[3] Curran D, Sahmoud T, Therasse P, et al. Prognostic factors in patients with pleural mesothelioma: The European Organization for Research and Treatment of Cancer experience. Journal of Clinical Oncology. 1998;**16**:145-152

[4] Zellos L, Christiani DC. Epidemiology, biologic behavior, and natural history of mesothelioma. Thoracic Surgery Clinics. 2004;**14**:469-477

[5] van Meerbeeck JP, Damhuis R. Facts, rumours and speculations about the mesothelioma epidemic. Respirology. 2011;**16**(7):1018-1019

[6] Flores RM, Zakowski M, Venkatraman E, Krug L, Rosenzweig K, Dycoco J, et al. Prognostic factors in the treatment of malignant pleural mesothelioma at a large tertiary referral center. Journal of Thoracic Oncology. 2007;**2**(10):957-965

[7] Sugarbaker DJ, Flores RM, Jaklitsch MT, et al. Resection margins, extrapleural nodal status, and cell type determine postoperative long-term survival in trimodality therapy of malignant pleural mesothelioma: Results in 183 patients. The Journal of Thoracic and Cardiovascular Surgery. 1999;**117**(1):54-63

[8] Sterman DH, Treat J, Litzky LA, et al. Adenovirus-mediated herpes simplex virus with thymidine kinase/ganciclovir gene therapy in patients with localized malignancy: Results of a phase I clinical trial in malignant mesothelioma. Human Gene Therapy. 1998;**9**(7):1083-1092

[9] Takita H, Dougherthy TJ. Intracavitary photodynamic therapy for malignant pleural mesothelioma. Seminars in Surgical Oncology. 1995;**11**(5):368-371

[10] Hendon JE, Green MR, Chahinian AP, et al. Factors predictive of survival among 337 patients with mesothelioma treated between 1984 and 1994 by the cancer and leukemia group B. Chest. 1998;**113**:723-731

[11] Pass HI. Biomarkers and prognostic factors for mesothelioma. Annals of Cardiothoracic Surgery. 2012;**1**(4):449-456

[12] Pass HI, Giroux D, Kennedy C, et al. IASLC staging committee and participating institutions. Supplementary prognostic variables for pleural mesothelioma: A report from the IASLC staging committee. Journal of Thoracic Oncology. 2014;**9**:856-864

[13] Edwards JG, Abrams KR, Leverment JN, Spyt TJ, Waller DA, O'Byrne KJ. Prognostic factors for malignant mesothelioma in 142 patients: Validation of CALGB and EORTC prognostic scoring systems. Thorax. 2000;**55**(9):731-735

[14] Steele JP, Rudd RM. Malignant mesothelioma: Predictors of prognosis and clinical trials. Thorax. 2000;**55**(9):725-726

[15] Van Gerwen M, Alpert N, Wolf A, et al. Prognostic factors of survival in patients with malignant pleural mesothelioma: An analysis of the National Cancer Database. Carcinogenesis. 2019;**40**(4):529-536

[16] van Zandwijk N, Clarke C, Henderson D, et al. Guidelines for the diagnosis and treatment of malignant pleural mesothelioma. Journal of Thoracic Disease. 2013;**5**(6):E254-E307

[17] Nowak AK, Francis RJ, Phillips MJ, et al. A novel prognostic model for malignant mesothelioma incorporating quantitative FDG-PET imaging with clinical parameters. Clinical Cancer Research. 2010;**16**(8):2409-2417

[18] Zhuo Y, Lin L, Zhang M. Pretreatment thrombocytosis as a significant prognostic factor in malignant mesothelioma: A meta-analysis. Platelets. 2016;**28**(6):560-566

[19] Yao ZH, Tian GY, Yang SX, et al. Serum albumin as a significant prognostic factor in patients with malignant pleural mesothelioma. Tumour Biology. 2014;**35**:6839-6845

[20] Yin W, Zheng G, Yang K, Song H, Liang Y. Analysis of prognostic factors of patients with malignant peritoneal mesothelioma. World Journal of Surgical Oncology. 2018;**16**(1)

[21] Zhuo Y, Lin L, Wei S, Zhang M. Pretreatment elevated serum lactate dehydrogenase as a significant prognostic factor in malignant mesothelioma. Medicine. 2016; **95**(52):e5706

[22] Abdel-Rahman O. Challenging a dogma; AJCC 8th staging system is not sufficient to predict outcomes of patients with malignant pleural mesothelioma. Lung Cancer. 2017;**113**:128-133

[23] Berzenji L, Van Schil P, Carp L. The eighth TNM classification for malignant pleural mesothelioma. Translational Lung Cancer Research. 2018;7(5):543-549

[24] Kawashima A, Libshitz HI. Malignant pleural mesothelioma: Manifestations in 50 cases. American Journal of Roentgenology. 1990;**155**:965-969

[25] Heelan RT, Rusch VW, Begg CB, et al. Staging of malignant pleural mesothelioma: Comparison of CT and MR imaging. American Journal of Roentgenology. 1999;**172**:1039-1047

[26] Armato SG, Ogarek JL, Starkey A, et al. Variability in mesothelioma tumor response classification. American Journal of Roentgenology. 2006;**186**:1000-1006

[27] Gill RR, Richards WG, Yeap BY, et al. Epithelial malignant pleural mesothelioma after extrapleural pneumonectomy: Stratification of survival with CT-derived tumor volume. American Journal of Roentgenology. 2012;**198**(2):359-363

[28] Flores RM, Riedel E, Donington JS, et al. Frequency of use and predictors of cancer-directed surgery in the management of malignant pleural mesothelioma in a community-based (surveillance, epidemiology, and end results [SEER]) population. Journal of Thoracic Oncology. 2010;**5**:1649-1654

[29] Spirtas R, Conelly RR, Tucker MA. Survival patterns for malignant mesothelioma: The SEER experience. International Journal of Cancer. 1988;**41**:525-530

[30] Milano MT, Zhang H. Malignant pleural mesothelioma: A population-based study of survival. Journal of Thoracic Oncology. 2010;**5**:1841-1848

[31] Taioli E, Wolf AS, Camacho-Rivera M, Flores RM. Women with malignant pleural mesothelioma have a threefold better survival rate than men. The Annals of Thoracic Surgery. 2014;**98**:1020-1024

[32] Wolf AS, Richards WG, Tilleman TR, et al. Characteristics of malignant pleural mesothelioma

in women. The Annals of Thoracic Surgery. 2010;**90**:949-956

[33] Rusch VW, Venkatraman ES. Important prognostic factors in patients with malignant pleural mesothelioma, managed surgically. The Annals of Thoracic Surgery. 1999;**68**:1799-1804

[34] Yan TD, Popa E, Brun EA, Cerruto CA, Sugarbaker PH. Sex difference in diffuse malignant peritoneal mesothelioma. The British Journal of Surgery. 2006;**93**:1536-1542

[35] Hillerdal G. Mesothelioma: Cases associated with non-occupational and low dose exposures. Occupational and Environmental Medicine. 1999;**56**:505-513

[36] Pinton G, Brunelli E, Murer B, et al. Estrogen receptor-beta affects the prognosis of human malignant mesothelioma. Cancer Research. 2009;**69**:4598-4604

[37] Rodríguez-Cid J, García-Acevedo O, Benjamin-Contreras J, et al. Expression of estrogen receptor beta (ERβ) and its prognostic value in pleural mesothelioma. Journal of Thoracic Disease. 2019;**11**(4):1456-1464

[38] Hassan R, Morrow B, Walsh T, et al. Inherited predisposition to malignant mesothelioma (MM) due to mutations in DNA repair genes. Journal of Clinical Oncology. 2018;**15**:8504-8504

[39] Panou V, Gadiraju M, Wolin A, et al. Frequency of germline mutations in cancer susceptibility genes in malignant mesothelioma. Journal of Clinical Oncology. 2018;**36**:2863-2871

[40] Pastorino S, Yoshikawa Y, Pass H, et al. A subset of mesotheliomas with improved survival occurring in carriers of BAP1 and other germline mutations. Journal of Clinical Oncology. 2018;**36**(35):3485-3494

[41] De Rienzo A, Archer MA, Yeap BY, et al. Gender-specific molecular and clinical features underlie malignant pleural mesothelioma. Cancer Research. 2016;**76**:319-328

[42] Pinton G, Moro L. Expression and therapeutic significance of estrogen receptor beta in malignant pleural mesothelioma. Future Science OA. 2017;**3**:Fso175

[43] Pinton G, Thomas W, Bellini P, et al. Estrogen receptor beta exerts tumor repressive functions in human malignant pleural mesothelioma via EGFR inactivation and affects response to gefitinib. PLoS One. 2010;**5**:e14110

[44] Jain S, Harris J, Ware J. Platelets: Linking hemostasis and cancer. Arteriosclerosis, Thrombosis, and Vascular Biology. 2010;**30**(12):2362-2367

[45] Honn KV, Tang DG, Crissman JD. Platelets and cancer metastasis: A causal relationship? Cancer and Metastasis Reviews. 1992;**11**(3-4):325-351

[46] Li N. Platelets in cancer metastasis: To help the "villain" to do evil. International Journal of Cancer. 2016;**138**(9):2078-2087

[47] Mezouar S, Mege D, Darbousset R, Farge D, Debourdeau P, Dignat-George F, et al. Involvement of platelet-derived microparticles in tumor progression and thrombosis. Seminars in Oncology. 2014;**41**(3):346-358

[48] Rolli M, Fransvea E, Pilch J, Saven A, Felding-Habermann B. Activated integrin alphavbeta3 cooperates with metalloproteinase MMP-9 in regulating migration of metastatic breast cancer cells. Proceedings of the National Academy of Sciences of the United States of America. 2003;**100**(16):9482-9487

[49] Deryugina EI, Quigley JP. Matrix metalloproteinases and tumor metastasis. Cancer Metastasis Reviews. 2006;**25**(1):9-34

[50] Sabrkhany S, Griffioen AW, Oude Egbrink MG. The role of blood platelets in tumor angiogenesis. Biochimica et Biophysica Acta. 2011;**1815**(2):189-196

[51] Kisucka J, Butterfield CE, Duda DG, Eichenberger SC, Saffaripour S, Ware J, et al. Platelets and platelet adhesion support angiogenesis while preventing excessive hemorrhage. Proceedings of the National Academy of Sciences of the United States of America. 2006;**103**(4):855-860

[52] Massberg S, Konrad I, Schurzinger K, Lorenz M, Schneider S, Zohlnhoefer D, et al. Platelets secrete stromal cell-derived factor 1alpha and recruit bone marrow-derived progenitor cells to arterial thrombi in vivo. The Journal of Experimental Medicine. 2006;**203**(5):1221-1233

[53] Borsig L, Wong R, Feramisco J, Nadeau DR, Varki NM, Varki A. Heparin and cancer revisited: Mechanistic connections involving platelets, P-selectin, carcinoma mucins, and tumor metastasis. Proceedings of the National Academy of Sciences of the United States of America. 2001;**98**(6):3352-3357

[54] Nieswandt B, Hafner M, Echtenacher B, Mannel DN. Lysis of tumor cells by natural killer cells in mice is impeded by platelets. Cancer Research. 1999;**59**(6):1295-1300

[55] Proctor MJ, Morrison DS, Talwar D, et al. A comparison of inflammation-based prognostic scores in patients with cancer. A Glasgow inflammation outcome study. European Journal of Cancer. 2011;**47**:2633-2641

[56] Urrejola GI, Bambs CE, Espinoza MA, et al. An elevated neutrophil/lymphocyte ratio is associated with poor prognosis in stage II resected colon cancer. Revista Médica de Chile. 2013;**141**:602-608

[57] Ozdemir Y, Akin ML, Sucullu I, Balta AZ, Yucel E. Pretreatment neutrophil/ lymphocyte ratio as a prognostic aid in colorectal cancer. Asian Pacific Journal of Cancer Prevention. 2014;**15**:2647-2650

[58] Azab B, Shah N, Radbel J, et al. Pretreatment neutrophil/lymphocyte ratio is superior to platelet/lymphocyte ratio as a predictor of long-term mortality in breast cancer patients. Medical Oncology. 2013;**30**:432-442

[59] Szkandera J, Absenger G, Liegl-Atzwanger B, et al. Elevated preoperative neutrophil/lymphocyte ratio is associated with poor prognosis in soft-tissue sarcoma patients. British Journal of Cancer. 2013;**108**:1677-1683

[60] Gondo T, Nakashima J, Ohno Y, et al. Prognostic value of neutrophil-to-lymphocyte ratio and establishment of novel preoperative risk stratification model in bladder cancer patients treated with radical cystectomy. Urology. 2012;**79**:1085-1091

[61] Tanrikulu AC, Abakay A, Kaplan MA, et al. A clinical, radiographic and laboratory evaluation of prognostic factors in 363 patients with malignant pleural mesothelioma. Respiration. 2010;**80**:480-487

[62] Nojiri S, Gemba K, Aoe K, et al. Survival and prognostic factors in malignant pleural mesothelioma: A retrospective study of 314 patients in the west part of Japan. Japanese Journal of Clinical Oncology. 2011;**41**:32-39

[63] Ghanim B, Hoda MA, Winter MP, et al. Pretreatment serum C-reactive protein levels predict benefit from multimodality treatment including

radical surgery in malignant pleural mesothelioma: A retrospective multicenter analysis. Annals of Surgery. 2012;**256**:357-362

[64] Morgan TM, Tang D, Stratton KL, et al. Preoperative nutritional status is an important predictor of survival in patients undergoing surgery for renal cell carcinoma. European Urology. 2011;**59**:923-928

[65] Nozoe T, Kohno M, Iguchi T, et al. The prognostic nutritional index can be a prognostic indicator in colorectal carcinoma. Surgery Today. 2012;**42**:532-535

[66] Nozoe T, Kimura Y, Ishida M, Saeki H, Korenaga D, Sugimachi K. Correlation of pre-operative nutritional condition with post-operative complications in surgical treatment for oesophageal carcinoma. European Journal of Surgical Oncology. 2002;**28**:396-400

[67] Murphy S, Probert G, Anderson J, et al. Malignant mesothelioma, hypoalbuminaemia and the effect of carboplatin/pemetrexed on survival. Clinical Oncology. 2013;**25**(12):713-718

[68] Hsu PP, Sabatini DM. Cancer cell metabolism: Warburg and beyond. Cell. 2008;**134**:703-707

[69] Serganova I, Rizwan A, Ni X, et al. Metabolic imaging: A link between lactate dehydrogenase A, lactate, and tumor phenotype. Clinical Cancer Research. 2011;**17**:6250-6261

[70] Metintas M, Metintas S, Ucgun I, et al. Prognostic factors in diffuse malignant pleural mesothelioma: Effects of pretreatment clinical and laboratory characteristics. Respiratory Medicine. 2001;**95**:829-835

[71] Ak G, Metintas S, Metintas M, et al. Prognostic factors according to the treatment schedule in malignant pleural mesothelioma. Journal of Thoracic Oncology. 2009;**4**:1425-1430

[72] Suzuki H, Hirashima T, Kobayashi M, et al. Prognostic factors in malignant pleural mesothelioma: A retrospective study. Internal Medicine. 2012;**51**:707-710

[73] Suzuki H, Asami K, Hirashima T, et al. Stratification of malignant pleural mesothelioma prognosis using recursive partitioning analysis. Lung. 2014;**192**:191-195

[74] Abakay O, Tanrikulu AC, Palanci Y, et al. The value of inflammatory parameters in the prognosis of malignant mesothelioma. The Journal of International Medical Research. 2014;**42**:554-565

[75] Kataoka Y, Yamamoto Y, Otsuki T, et al. A new prognostic index for overall survival in malignant pleural mesothelioma: The rPHS (regimen, PS, histology or stage) index. Japanese Journal of Clinical Oncology. 2015;**45**:562-568

[76] Vaupel P, Kallinowski F, Okunieff P. Blood flow, oxygen and nutrient supply, and metabolic microenvironment of human tumors: A review. Cancer Research. 1989;**49**:6449-6465

[77] Stubbs M, McSheehy PM, Griffiths JR, et al. Causes and consequences of tumour acidity and implications for treatment. Molecular Medicine Today. 2000;**6**:15-19

[78] Bonuccelli G, Tsirigos A, Whitaker-Menezes D, et al. Ketones and lactate "fuel" tumor growth and metastasis: Evidence that epithelial cancer cells use oxidative mitochondrial metabolism. Cell Cycle. 2010;**9**:3506-3514

[79] Martinez-Outschoorn UE, Prisco M, Ertel A, et al. Ketones and lactate

increase cancer cell "stemness," driving recurrence, metastasis and poor clinical outcome in breast cancer: Achieving personalized medicine via Metabolo-Genomics. Cell Cycle. 2011;**10**:1271-1286

[80] Nemoto S, Takeda K, Yu ZX, et al. Role for mitochondrial oxidants as regulators of cellular metabolism. Molecular and Cellular Biology. 2000;**20**:7311-7318

[81] Kolev Y, Uetake H, Takagi Y, et al. Lactate dehydrogenase-5 (LDH-5) expression in human gastric cancer: Association with hypoxia-inducible factor (HIF-1alpha) pathway, angiogenic factors production and poor prognosis. Annals of Surgical Oncology. 2008;**15**:2336-2344

[82] Rusch VW, Giroux D, Kennedy C, et al. Initial analysis of the International Association for the Study of Lung Cancer mesothelioma database. Journal of Thoracic Oncology. 2012;**7**:1631-1639

[83] Davidson B. Prognostic factors in malignant pleural mesothelioma. Human Pathology. 2015;**46**:789-804

[84] Kadota K, Suzuki K, Colovos C, et al. A nuclear grading system is a strong predictor of survival in epitheloid diffuse malignant pleural mesothelioma. Modern Pathology. 2012;**25**:260-271

[85] Galateau-Salle F, Churg A, Roggli V. Tumours of the pleura. Mesothelial tumours. Diffuse malignant mesothelioma. Epithelioid Mesothelioma. In: Travis WD, Brambilla E, Burke AP, Marx A, Nicholson AG, editors. The World Health Organisation Classification of Tumours of the Lung, Pleura, Thymus and Heart. 7th ed. Lyon, France: International Agency of Research on Cancer; 2015. pp. 156-164

[86] Habougit C, Thrombert-Paviot B, Karpathiou G, et al. Histopathologic features predict survival in diffuse pleural malignant mesothelioma on pleural biopsies. Virchows Archiv. 2017;**470**:639-646

[87] Gerdes J, Lemke H, Baisch H, et al. Cell cycle analysis of a cell proliferation-associated human nuclear antigen defined by the monoclonal antibody Ki-67. Journal of Immunology. 1984;**133**:1710-1715

[88] Verheijen R, Kuijpers HJ, Schlingemann RO, et al. Ki-67 detects a nuclear matrix-associated proliferation-related antigen. I. Intracellular localization during interphase. Journal of Cell Science. 1989;**92**(pt 1):123-130

[89] Dowsett M, Smith IE, Ebbs SR, et al. Prognostic value of Ki67 expression after short-term presurgical endocrine therapy for primary breast cancer. Journal of the National Cancer Institute. 2007;**99**:167-170

[90] Baum M, Budzar AU, Cuzick J, et al. Anastrozole alone or in combination with tamoxifen versus tamoxifen alone for adjuvant treatment of postmenopausal women with early breast cancer: First results of the ATAC randomised trial. Lancet. 2002;**359**:2131-2139

[91] Penault-Llorca F, Andre F, Sagan C, et al. Ki67 expression and docetaxel efficacy in patients with estrogen receptor-positive breast cancer. Journal of Clinical Oncology. 2009;**27**:2809-2815

[92] Orth JD, Tang Y, Shi J, et al. Quantitative live imaging of cancer and normal cells treated with Kinesin-5 inhibitors indicates significant differences in phenotypic responses and cell fate. Molecular Cancer Therapeutics. 2008;**7**:3480-3489

[93] Mitchison TJ. The proliferation rate paradox in antimitotic chemotherapy. Molecular Biology of the Cell. 2012;**23**:1-6

[94] Hirano H, Fujisawa T, Maekawa K, et al. Malignant mesothelioma of the peritoneum: Case reports and immunohistochemical findings including Ki-67 expression. Medical Molecular Morphology. 2010;**43**:53-59

[95] Pillai K, Pourgholami M, Chua T, Morris D. Prognostic significance of Ki67 expression in malignant peritoneal mesothelioma. American Journal of Clinical Oncology. 2015;**38**(4):388-394

[96] Kusamura S, Torres Mesa PA, Cabras A, et al. The role of Ki-67 and pre-cytoreduction parameters in selecting diffuse malignant peritoneal mesothelioma (DMPM) patients for cytoreductive surgery (CRS) and hyperthermic intraperitoneal chemotherapy (HIPEC). Annals of Surgical Oncology. 2016;**23**(5):1468-1473

[97] Ghanim B, Klikovits T, Hoda MA, et al. Ki67 index is an independent prognostic factor in epithelioid but not in non-epithelioid malignant pleural mesothelioma: A multicenter study. British Journal of Cancer. 2015;**112**(5):783-792

[98] Vigneri P, Martorana F, Manzella L, Stella S. Biomarkers and prognostic factors for malignant pleural mesothelioma. Future Oncology. 2015;**11**(24s):29-33

[99] Li D, Wang B, Long H, Wen F. Diagnostic accuracy of calretinin for malignant mesothelioma in serous effusions: A meta-analysis. Scientific Reports. 2015;**5**:9507

[100] Yukio T, Inai K, Ishikawa Y, et al. The trial of differentiation grading of epithelioid mesothelioma with reference to its clinicopathological significance. In: Kyoto: International Mesothelioma Interest Group Meeting. 2010. Abstr P10-1

[101] Kao SC, Klebe S, Henderson DW, et al. Low calretinin expression and high neutrophil-to-lymphocyte ratio are poor prognostic factors in patients with malignant mesothelioma undergoing extrapleural pneumonectomy. Journal of Thoracic Oncology. 2011;**6**:1923-1929

[102] Kao SC, Pavlakis N, Harvie R, et al. High blood neutrophil-to- lymphocyte ratio is an indicator of poor prognosis in malignant mesothelioma patients undergoing systemic therapy. Clinical Cancer Research. 2010;**16**:5805-5813

[103] Linton A, Pavlakis N, O'Connell R, et al. Factors associated with survival in a large series of patients with malignant pleural mesothelioma in New South Wales. British Journal of Cancer. 2014;**111**:1860-1869

[104] Thapa B, Walkiewicz M, Murone C, et al. Calretinin but not caveolin-1 correlates with tumour histology and survival in malignant mesothelioma. Pathology. 2016;**48**(7):660-665

[105] Robinson BW, Creaney J, Lake R, et al. Mesothelin-family proteins and diagnosis of mesothelioma. Lancet. 2003;**362**(9396):1612-1616

[106] Franko A, Dolzan V, Kovac V, Arneric N, Dodic-Fikfak M. Soluble mesothelin-related peptides levels in patients with malignant mesothelioma. Disease Markers. 2012;**32**:123-131

[107] Cristaudo A, Foddis R, Vivaldi A, et al. Clinical significance of serum mesothelin in patients with mesothelioma and lung cancer. Clinical Cancer Research. 2007;**13**:5076-5081

[108] Grigoriu BD, Scherpereel A, Devos P, et al. Utility of osteopontin and serum mesothelin in malignant pleural mesothelioma diagnosis and prognosis assessment. Clinical Cancer Research. 2007;**13**:2928-2935

[109] Creaney J, Francis RJ, Dick IM, et al. Serum soluble mesothelin concentrations in malignant pleural mesothelioma: Relationship to tumor volume, clinical stage and changes in tumor burden. Clinical Cancer Research. 2011;**17**:1181-1189

[110] Dipalma N, Luisi V, Di Serio F, et al. Biomarkers in malignant mesothelioma: Diagnostic and prognostic role of soluble mesothelin-related peptide. The International Journal of Biological Markers. 2011;**26**:160-165

[111] Schneider J, Hoffmann H, Dienemann H, Herth FJ, Meister M, Muley T. Diagnostic and prognostic value of soluble mesothelin-related proteins in patients with malignant pleural mesothelioma in comparison with benign asbestosis and lung cancer. Journal of Thoracic Oncology. 2008;**3**:1317-1324

[112] Creaney J, Yeoman D, Naumoff LK, et al. Soluble mesothelin in effusions: A useful tool for the diagnosis of malignant mesothelioma. Thorax. 2007;**62**:569-576

[113] Linch M, Gennatas S, Kazikin S, et al. A serum mesothelin level is a prognostic indicator for patients with malignant mesothelioma in routine clinical practice. BMC Cancer. 2014;**14**:674

[114] Creaney J, Dick IM, Meniawy TM, et al. Comparison of Fibulin-3 and mesothelin as markers in malignant mesothelioma. Thorax. 2014;**69**:895-902

[115] Tian L, Zeng R, Wang X, Shen C, Lai Y, Wang M, et al. Prognostic significance of soluble mesothelin in malignant pleural mesothelioma: A meta-analysis. Oncotarget. 2017;**8**(28)

[116] Timpl R, Sasaki T, Kostka G, Chu ML. Fibulins: A versatile family of extracellular matrix proteins. Nature Reviews. Molecular Cell Biology. 2003;**4**:479-489

[117] Kobayashi N, Kostka G, Garbe JH, et al. A comparative analysis of the bulin protein family. Biochemical characterization, binding interactions, and tissue localization. The Journal of Biological Chemistry. 2007;**282**:11805-11816

[118] Kirschner MB, Pulford E, Hoda MA, et al. Fibulin-3 levels in malignant pleural mesothelioma are associated with prognosis but not diagnosis. British Journal of Cancer. 2015;**113**:963-969

[119] Hooper CE, Lyburn ID, Searle J, Darby M, et al. The south west area mesothelioma and pemetrexed trial: A multicentre prospective observational study evaluating novel markers of chemotherapy response and prognostication. British Journal of Cancer. 2015;**112**:1175-1182

[120] Pass HI, Levin SM, Harbut MR, et al. Fibulin-3 as a blood and effusion biomarker for pleural mesothelioma. The New England Journal of Medicine. 2012;**367**(15):1417-1427

[121] Anborgh PH, Wilson SM, Tuck AB, et al. New dual monoclonal ELISA for measuring plasma osteopontin as a biomarker associated with survival in prostate cancer: Clinical validation and comparison of multiple ELISAs. Clinical Chemistry. 2009;**55**(5):895-903

[122] Pass H, Goparaju C, Espin-Garcia O, Donington J, et al. Plasma biomarker enrichment of clinical prognostic indices in malignant pleural mesothelioma. Journal of Thoracic Oncology. 2016;**11**(6):900-909

[123] Kawabat SE, Bast RC, Bhan AK, Welch WR, Knapp RC, Colvi RB. Tissue distribution of a coelomic epithelium

related antigen recognized by the monoclonal antibody 0025. International Journal of Gynecology. 1984;**2**:275-285

[124] Bast RC, Klug TL, John E, et al. A radioimmunoassay using a mono clonal antibody to monitor the course of epithelial ovarian cancer. The New England Journal of Medicine. 1983;**309**:883-887

[125] Koclma IA, Nap M, Rodenburg CJ, Fleuren GJ. The value of tumour marker CA125 in surgical pathology. Histopathology. 1987;**11**:287-294

[126] Berardi R, Fiordoliva I, De Lisa M, Ballatore Z, Caramanti M, Morgese F, et al. Clinical and pathologic predictors of clinical outcome of malignant pleural mesothelioma. Tumori. 2016;**102**(2):190-195

[127] Duan HJ, Itoh N, Yamagami O, Katsuyama T, Shigematsu H. Diffuse malignant mesothelioma in a young woman with high serum level of CA125. Acta Pathologica Japonica. 1991;**41**:158-163

[128] Simsek H, Kadayifci A, Okan E. Importance of serum CA 125 levels in malignant peritoneal mesothelioma. Tumor Biology. 1996;**17**(1):1-4

[129] Francart J, Vaes E, Henrard S, et al. A prognostic index for progression-free survival in malignant mesothelioma with application to the design of phase II trials: A combined analysis of 10 EORTC trials. European Journal of Cancer. 2009;**45**(13):2304-2315

[130] Blayney JK, Ceresoli GL, Castagneto B, et al. Response to chemotherapy is predictive in relation to longer overall survival in an individual patient combined-analysis with pleural mesothelioma. European Journal of Cancer. 2012;**48**:2983-2992

[131] Billé A, Krug L, Woo K, Rusch V, Zauderer M. Contemporary analysis of prognostic factors in patients with unresectable malignant pleural mesothelioma. Journal of Thoracic Oncology. 2016;**11**(2):249-255

[132] Larson SM, Erdi Y, Akhurst T, et al. Tumor treatment response based on visual and quantitative changes in global tumor glycolysis using PET-FDG imaging. The visual response score and the change in total lesion glycolysis. Clinical Positron Imaging. 1999;**2**(3):159-171

[133] Ceresoli G, Chiti A, Zucali P, et al. Early evaluation in malignant pleural mesothelioma by positron emission tomography with [^{18}F] fluorodeoxyglucose. Journal of Clinical Oncology. 2006;**24**:4587-4593

[134] Francis R, Byrne M, van der Schaaf A, et al. Early prediction of response to chemotherapy and survival in malignant pleural mesothelioma using a novel semiautomated 3-dimensional volume-based analysis of serial ^{18}F-FDG PET scans. Journal of Nuclear Medicine. 2007;**48**:1449-1458

[135] Chung MK, Jeong HS, Park SG, et al. Metabolic tumor volume of ^{18}Fluorodeoxyglucose positron emission tomography/computed tomography predicts short-term outcome to radiotherapy with or without chemotherapy in pharyngeal cancer. Clinical Cancer Research. 2009;**15**(18):5861-5868

[136] Veit-Haibach P, Schaefer N, Steinert H, et al. Combined FDG-PET/CT in response evaluation of malignant pleural mesothelioma. Lung Cancer. 2010;**67**:311-317

[137] Lee H, Hyun S, Lee K, et al. Volume-based parameter of ^{18}F-FDG PET/CT in malignant pleural mesothelioma: Prediction of therapeutic response and prognostic implications. Annals of Surgical Oncology. 2010;**17**:2787-2794

[138] Basu S, Saboury B, Torigian DA, et al. Current evidence base of FDG-PET/CT imaging in the clinical management of malignant pleural mesothelioma: Emerging significance of image segmentation and global disease assessment. Molecular Imaging and Biology. 2011;**13**(5):801-811

[139] Genestreti G, Moretti A, Piciucchi S, et al. FDG PET/CT response evaluation in malignant pleural mesothelioma patients treated with talc pleurodesis and chemotherapy. Journal of Cancer. 2012;**3**:241-245

[140] Schaefer N, Veit-Haibach P, Soyka J, Steinert H, Stahel R. Continued pemetrexed and platin-based chemotherapy in patients with malignant pleural mesothelioma (MPM): Value of ^{18}F-FDGPET/CT. European Journal of Radiology. 2012;**81**:e19-e25

[141] Klabatsa A, Chicklore S, Barrington S, Goh V, Lang-Lazdunski L, Cook C. The association of ^{18}F-FDG PET/CT parameters with survival in malignant pleural mesothelioma. European Journal of Nuclear Medicine and Molecular Imaging. 2014;**41**:276-282

[142] Marin-Oyaga VA, Salavati A, Houshmand S, et al. Feasibility and performance of an adaptive contrast-oriented FDG PET/CT quantification technique for global disease assessment of malignant pleural mesothelioma and a brief review of the literature. Hellenic Journal of Nuclear Medicine. 2015;**18**(1):11-18

[143] Zucali P, Lopci E, Ceresoli G, et al. Prognostic and predictive role of [^{18}F]fluorodeoxyglucose positron emission tomography (FDG-PET) in patients with unresectable malignant pleural mesothelioma (MPM) treated with up-front pemetrexed-based chemotherapy. Cancer Medicine. 2017;**6**(10):2287-2296

[144] Niccoli-Asabella A, Di Palo A, Altini C, et al. ^{18}F-FDG PET/CT in therapy response and in predicting responders or non-responders in malignant pleural mesothelioma patients, by using semi-quantitative mRECIST and EORTC criteria. Hellenic Journal of Nuclear Medicine. 2018;**21**(3):191-197

[145] Luo W, Rao M, Qu J, Luo D. Applications of liquid biopsy in lung cancer—Diagnosis, prognosis prediction, and disease monitoring. American Journal of Translational Research. 2018;**10**(12):3911-3923

[146] Cavallari I, Urso L, Sharova E, Pasello G, Ciminale V. Liquid biopsy in malignant pleural mesothelioma: State of the art, pitfalls, and perspectives. Frontiers in Oncology. 2019;**9**:7-10

[147] Khanna S, Thomas A, Abate-Daga D, et al. Malignant mesothelioma effusions are infiltrated by CD3+ T cells highly expressing PD-L1 and the PD-L1+ tumor cells within these effusions are susceptible to ADCC by the anti-PD-L1 antibody avelumab. Journal of Thoracic Oncology. 2016;**11**(11):1993-2005

[148] Combaz-Lair C, Galateau-Salle F, McLeer-Florin A, et al. Immune biomarkers PD-1/PD-L1 and TLR3 in malignant pleural mesotheliomas. Human Pathology. 2016;**52**:9-18

[149] Cedres S, Ponce-Aix S, Zugazagoitia J, et al. Analysis of expression of programmed cell death 1 ligand 1 (PD-L1) in malignant pleural mesothelioma (MPM). PLoS One. 2015;**10**(3):e0121071

[150] Garon EB, Rizvi NA, Hui R, et al. Pembrolizumab for the treatment of non-small-cell lung cancer. The New England Journal of Medicine. 2015;**372**(21):2018-2028

[151] Topalian SL, Hodi FS, Brahmer JR, et al. Safety, activity, and

immunecorrelates of anti-PD-1 antibody in cancer. The New England Journal of Medicine. 2012;**366**(26):2443-2454

[152] Valmary-Degano S, Colpart P, Villeneuve L, et al. Immunohistochemical evaluation of two antibodies against PD-L1 and prognostic significance of PD-L1 expression in epithelioid peritoneal malignant mesothelioma: A RENAPE study. European Journal of Surgical Oncology. 2017;**43**(10):1915-1923

[153] Levallet G, Vaisse-Lesteven M, Le Stang N, et al. Plasma cell membrane localization of c-MET predicts longer survival in patients with malignant mesothelioma: A series of 157 cases from the MESOPATH group. Journal of Thoracic Oncology. 2012;**7**(3):599-606

[154] Zucali PA, Giovannetti E, Destro A, et al. Thymidylate synthase and excision repair cross-complementing group-1 as predictors of responsiveness in mesothelioma patients treated with pemetrexed/carboplatin. Clinical Cancer Research. 2011;**17**(8):2581-2590

[155] Henderson DW, Reid G, Kao SC, van Zandwijk N, Klebe S. Challenges and controversies in the diagnosis of malignant mesothelioma: Part 2. Malignant mesothelioma subtypes, pleural synovial sarcoma, molecular and prognostic aspects of mesothelioma, BAP1, aquaporin-1 and microRNA. Journal of Clinical Pathology. 2013;**66**:854-861

[156] Zhou J, Zhong H, Zhang J, Jin S, Roudi R, Ma H. Development and validation of a prognostic signature for malignant pleural mesothelioma. Frontiers in Oncology. 2019;**9**:6-9

Chapter 6

Biomarkers Progress and Therapeutic Implications in Malignant Mesothelioma

Jordyn Feinstein and Muaiad Kittaneh

Abstract

We are witnessing enormous efforts to identify prognostic and predictive biomarkers to inform treatment decisions in malignant mesothelioma. In this chapter, we will review and discuss the current literature and supportive evidence for the progress in development and use of biomarkers in malignant mesothelioma. There are currently several clinical trials evaluating treatment options in mesothelioma, and this will be an up-to-date review of these trials from published literature.

Keywords: mesothelioma, biomarkers, ASS1, BAP1, CDKN2A, mesothelin, NF-2, PDL-1, VEGF, WT-1

1. Epidemiology of mesothelioma

Malignant mesothelioma (MM) is an aggressive, rare cancer of pleural (80%), and peritoneal cells and less frequently in the pericardium and tunica vaginalis of the testis. MM has historically been linked to mineral fiber exposure. Asbestos is a collective term given to six mineral fibers including actinolite, amosite, anthophyllite, chrysotile, crocidolite, and tremolite [1]. Exposure to other non-asbestos mineral fibers including erionite and fluoro-edenite has also been linked to MM [2]. However, cases of MM have been found in patients who were not exposed to these mineral fibers. This led researchers to discover other epidemiologies of mesothelioma heavily linked to genetic mutations, including tumor suppressors like BRCA1-associated protein (BAP1) [3].

2. Biomarkers in mesothelioma

Recent research has been aimed at studying various biomarkers in malignant mesothelioma. Researchers hope that by identifying and studying specific biomarkers, new therapies can be developed that better target the unique pathways of malignant mesothelioma pathogenesis.

2.1 Vascular endothelial growth factor

The VEGF pathway is believed to play a critical role in angiogenesis and lymphangiogenesis in human malignant mesothelioma tumors [4]. In one study, more than 95% of malignant pleural mesothelioma (MPM) samples stained positive for VEGF [5]. An increase expression of VEGF was specifically observed in the epithelioid histology, more than biphasic and sarcomatoid. VEGF was not felt to have any prognostic significance in this study [5]. In another study, VEGF was found to be an independent, poor prognostic factor in MPM [6]. The phase III MAPS study showed that the addition of bevacizumab, a humanized anti-VEGF monoclonal IgG1 antibody, to frontline cisplatin/pemetrexed in unresectable malignant pleural mesothelioma improves overall survival (18.8 vs. 16.1; hazard ratio 0.77 [0.62–0.95]; p = 0.0167) compared to cisplatin/pemetrexed alone regardless of tumor histology [7]. Analysis from the MAPS study showed that high VEGF concentrations were associated with worse progression free survival and overall survival but VEGF did not have a clinically meaningful predictive significance of response to bevacizumab [8]. Other antiangiogenic agents like Sorafenib and axitinib have showed limited activity in malignant mesotheliomas [9, 10]. Ramucirumab is a recombinant human immunoglobulin G1 monoclonal antibody that binds to the extracellular domain of VEGFR-2 and prevents the binding of VEGFR ligands: VEGF-A, VEGF-C, and VEGF-D. A recently published Phase II abstract showed that the addition of Ramucirumab to gemcitabine significantly improved the overall survival in advanced MPM patients who progressed on first-line platinum-pemetrexed chemotherapy. This was observed regardless of patient age, tumor stage (locally advanced vs. metastatic), histotype (epithelioid vs. non-epithelioid), and time to progression at the first-line treatment [11].

2.2 Arginosuccinate synthetase

Certain cancer cells have a higher nutritional demand compared to normal cells. Arginine is an amino acid that plays an important role in biological and signaling pathways [12]. Arginine is either synthesized in the body or consumed in the diet. Normal cells synthesize arginine through the urea cycle. Research suggests that certain cancer cells cannot internally make arginine because they lack the urea cycle enzyme argininosuccinate synthetase 1 (ASS1) which ultimately makes them dependent on exogenous supplies of arginine, an important amino acid for cancer survival and growth [13]. ASS is a key enzyme that converts citrulline to arginine. This has led scientists to hypothesize that targeting the arginine synthesis pathway may be an effective therapeutic approach that targets cancer cells and spares normal cells.

Mesothelioma is one of the tumors that usually does not express ASS [14]. Arginine degradation is dependent on different enzymes, including an enzyme called arginine deiminase (ADI) that degrades arginine to citrulline. In turn, citrulline can be recycled back to arginine in normal cells through ASS [14]. A pegylated arginine deiminase (ADI-PEG 20) has been developed as an arginine depleting agent and is currently being tested in a randomized, double-blind, phase 2/3 study in subjects with malignant pleural mesothelioma with low argininosuccinate synthetase 1 expression to assess ADI-PEG 20 with pemetrexed and cisplatin (Clinicaltrials.gov ID NCT02709512).

2.3 Aurora kinase

Aurora kinase gene expression is upregulated in mesothelioma tumor tissue and is considered a negative prognostic factor [15–17]. The Aurora proteins are serine/threonine kinases that function in various stages of mitosis. Aurora kinase proteins A/B play an important role in mitosis, monopolar spindles formation, chromosomal segregation cytokinesis, and polyploidy. These proteins are overexpressed in mesothelioma [18]. Aurora kinase inhibitors, like ZM447439, are able to inhibit cell growth in all mesothelioma cell lines [18]. Alisertib (MLN8237) is a selective aurora kinase A inhibitor that is currently being evaluated in pretreated patients with unresectable MPM (Clinicaltrials.gov NCT02293005).

2.4 Wilms' tumor protein

WT-1 is a zinc finger transcription factor protein that is responsible for controlling the expression of genes involved in cellular growth, differentiation, and/or apoptosis [19]. WT1 is a nuclear protein that is processed and highly overexpressed on the cell surface of MPM. Immunohistochemical (IHC) staining for WT1 is routinely used in establishing the diagnosis of mesothelioma. WT-1 protein expression is detected by IHC in 78.1% of MPM and associated with improved overall survival and prognosis [20]. Although WT1 protein is expressed on the cell surface in the context of MHC molecules, which makes it a target for T-cell based immunotherapeutic approach [21]. A randomized phase II trial of adjuvant galinpepimut-S, WT-1 analogue peptide vaccine, after multimodality therapy for patients with WT-1 + MPM showed that a favorable safety profile with suggested improvement in progression-free survival and overall survival and a larger randomized trial is planned [22].

2.5 Mesothelin

Mesothelin is a tumor differentiation protein that is normally expressed in low amounts on the pleural, peritoneal, and pericardial mesothelial cells. Mesothelin is highly expressed in malignant mesothelioma as well as other cancers like pancreatic, ovarian, and lung adenocarcinoma [23–25]. The differential expression of mesothelin between normal tissues and malignant cells made it an attractive candidate for cancer therapy. Mesothelin targeting agents including chimeric antigen receptor (CAR) T cells and vaccination strategies are currently in development for the treatment of MPM. CRS-207 is a live-attenuated strain of the bacterium *Listeria monocytogenes* that is engineered to express mesothelin. CRS-207 induces antitumor immune responses and increase the susceptibility of neoplastic cells to immune-mediated killing. A phase I study combining CRS-207 and pemetrexed/cisplatin chemotherapy induced significant changes in the local tumor microenvironment and objective tumor responses in a majority of treated patients [26].

2.6 Programmed death-receptor ligand

PD-L1 is overexpressed in 40–50% of mesothelioma and associated with poor outcome. In one study, high PD-L1 expression was associated with non-epithelioid MM, poor clinical outcome, and increased immunological infiltrates [27]. Several PD-L1 and PD1 targeting agents have been studied in mesothelioma with modest activity. Pembrolizumab, nivolumab, and ipilimumab are routinely used in the second-line therapy of malignant mesothelioma. PD-L1 testing is not required for prescribing pembrolizumab or nivolumab in the second-line therapy for patients with PMP [28]. Limited data suggests that high PD-L1 expression (≥25% positive tumor cells) seems to be a predictor of higher overall response rate to nivolumab on nivolumab plus ipilimumab and even better objective response rate when the PD-L1 expression is >50% [29]. Real-world data suggests that the high PD-L1 expression (≥50%) and non-epithelioid histology are associated with an improved objective response rate to pembrolizumab compared to intermediate (5–49%) and negative PD-L1 expression (<5%) in the second-line therapy of MPM [30].

2.7 BRCA1-associated protein

BRCA1-associated protein (BAP1) is a powerful deubiquitylating enzyme that acts to suppress the tumor growth. This means that it removes ubiquitin tags from specific proteins to modify and regulate their function or interaction with other molecules. BAP1 has been shown to have different tumor-suppressing functions when localized to the nucleus vs. cytoplasm. In the nucleus, it is promoted to double-stranded DNA break sites to aid in repair via homologous recombination, therefore inhibiting the growth of the damaged, mutated DNA [31, 32]. In the cytoplasm, BAP1 deubiquitylates type-3 inositol-1,4,5-trisphosphate-receptor (IP3R3) on the endoplasmic reticulum (ER). Once stabilized, IP3R3 allows the efflux of calcium (Ca^{2+}) from the ER into the cytoplasm. This increase in Ca^{2+} promotes cytochrome c activation and induces cell apoptosis [32, 33]. More recently, it has been proposed that BAP1 also regulates ferroptosis, an iron-dependent programmed cell death via the repression of cystine transporter SLC7A11 [34].

Somatic inactivating mutations in *BAP1* have been associated with numerous malignancies including female reproductive cancers, uveal melanoma, renal cell carcinoma, pancreatic cancer, and leukemia [35–41]. Somatic mutations in *BAP1* were also initially reported in up to 23% of MPM [42]. These results were reproduced in various studies with *BAP1* loss ranging from 20 to 60% in MM, further exemplifying its major role in the development of malignancy [35, 43–45].

Germline mutations in *BAP1* are associated with a novel cancer syndrome named "BAP1 Cancer Syndrome." This syndrome infers increased susceptibility to a variety of malignancies including mesothelioma, uveal and skin melanoma, cholangiocarcinoma, renal cell, basal cell, and squamous cell carcinomas, among others [32]. Malignant mesotheliomas that develop in BAP1 germline mutation carriers tend to be less aggressive with better prognosis and improved survival compared to sporadic mesothelioma [46].

There are currently no standard therapeutic approach for *BAP1* loss in mesothelioma. Histone deacetylase (HDAC) inhibitors reversed the H2A hyperubiquitination caused by *BAP1* loss, and they shift the gene expression profile of class 2 cells toward a class 1 profile in a UVM cell line [47, 48]. A phase 3 study comparing vorinostat (an HDAC inhibitor) with placebo in relapsed or refractory MPM concluded vorinostat did not improve overall survival compared to placebo and led to a statistically significant but not clinically relevant improvement in PFS [48, 49]. Molecular analysis to detect *BAP1* mutations in patients treated on this study has not been reported [48, 49].

BAP1 loss leads to increased expression of enhancer of zeste homolog 2 (EZH2) protein [50]. EZH2 is a protein component of the polycomb repressive complex 2 (PRC2) enzyme involved in chromatin modification [51]. Analysis of The Cancer Genome Atlas (TCGA) data revealed that EZH2 mRNA expression was increased in mesothelioma tumor samples [50]. Silencing EZH2 induced the apoptosis in *BAP1*-mutant mesothelioma cell lines [50]. EZH2 inhibition also reduced the mesothelioma tumor size in *BAP1*-mutant mice [50]. By contrast, Schoumacher and colleagues showed that EZH2 was not overexpressed in UM cases, and subsequently, UM cases with BAP1 loss were insensitive to the EZH2 inhibitor, EPZ-6438 [52]. These findings highlight the tissue-dependent expression of epigenetic regulators and differing roles in carcinogenesis. Tazemetostat (an EZH2 inhibitor) has been tested in mesothelioma patients with BAP1 loss-of-function and showed some promising activity. The disease control of tazemetostat was 47% at 12 weeks and 25% of patients-maintained disease control at 24 weeks [53].

PARP inhibition is another potential targeted therapy option in patients with somatic or germline *BAP1* mutations. Clinical trials are underway to investigate the role of PARP inhibitors in patients with DNA-repair protein defects, including BAP1. Currently there is a trial investigating niraparib (PARP inhibitor) (Clinicaltrials.gov ID NCT03207347) and three trials investigating olaparib (another PARP inhibitor) in BAP1 and other DDR deficient neoplasms (Clinicaltrials.gov ID NCT03786796, NCT03531840, NCT03375307). Combination therapies using nivolumab in combination with talazoparib in unresectable or metastatic melanoma patients with mutations in BRCA or BRCAness are also underway (NCT03531840).

A recent study published by Hassan et al. suggested that patients with pleural mesothelioma with loss-of-function mutations in *BAP1* and other DNA repair genes appeared to benefit from platinum chemotherapy compared with patients without inherited mutations [54].

2.8 Neurofibromatosis type 2

Neurofibromatosis type 2 (NF2) is another tumor suppressor gene most commonly associated with the disorder Neurofibromatosis 2, in which malignancies including vestibular schwannomas and meningiomas are common. However, in more recent years, the somatic mutations of NF2 have been linked to malignant mesothelioma, in addition to multiple other organ systems [55–57]. *NF2* gene is somatically mutated in 40–50% of MPM [57–59]. *NF2* encodes for a multifunctional protein named merlin which regulates the hippo signaling pathway among other pathways related to tumor progression and oncogenic activity [56, 60]. Disruption of the *NF2* tumor suppressor gene by mutation and/or deletion results in lack of expression of the functional merlin protein [61]. Merlin is a protein that regulates cellular cytoskeleton dynamic through its function as a linker between membrane proteins and the actin cytoskeleton. Merlin is involved in cell communication, adhesion, and motility, which are functions that are related to the invasive properties of malignant cells [62]. Merlin exerts its effect through forming a complex with the cytoplasmic kinase protein focal adhesion kinase (FAK) controlling cell adhesion, migration, and invasion through integrating signals from growth factor receptors and integrins [63–65]. Merlin inactivation is a critical step in MM pathogenesis and is related, at least in part, to upregulation of FAK activity. Merlin attenuates FAK phosphorylation and disrupt the interaction of FAK with its binding partners Src and p85, the regulatory subunit of Pi3K [58]. FAK expression and/or activity are reported to be upregulated in a wide range of malignancies including mesothelioma [62].

Loss of merlin, a product of the neurofibromatosis 2 tumor suppressor gene is being evaluated as a biomarker for FAK inhibitor sensitivity in mesothelioma. When NF2 is absent or inactivated, these regulation pathways are disrupted which result in the constitutive activation of oncogenesis [56]. Interestingly, when NF2 is reactivated and expressed in mesothelioma cells, invasiveness regresses [62]. Targeting NF2 or downstream proteins like FAK has become an attractive therapeutic strategy in mesothelioma. Defactinib (VS-6063) is a FAK inhibitor. Merlin-low mesothelioma cell lines are more sensitive to defactinib than merlin-high cell lines in vitro and in vivo [62].

Defactinib (VS-6063) has been evaluated as a single agent in MPM. The phase II COMMAND trial was a randomized, placebo-controlled phase II study of defactinib in patients with unresectable mesothelioma who had had a stable disease or a PR following at least 4 cycles of platinum-based pemetrexed. Patients were randomized to receive maintenance defactinib or placebo. Patients were stratified by tumor merlin immunohistochemistry status (high vs. low) prior to randomization, and the study aimed to measure the effect of treatment allocation on the overall survival and progression-free survival. The study showed no difference in the progression-free survival or overall survival between the two treatment arms in the intent-to-treat population or in patients who had merlin-low tumors [66]. Defactinib is currently being evaluated in combination with pembrolizumab in patients with pleural mesothelioma (Clinicaltrials.gov NCT04201145).

Another therapeutic approach that is currently being evaluated in NF2 mutant MM is NEDD8 activating enzyme (NAE) inhibition. Merlin is a negative regulator of mTORC1 and the loss of Merlin results in constitutive activation of the mTORC pathway [67, 68]. The exact mechanism by which Merlin suppresses mTOR signaling is unknown.

Merlin also suppresses tumorigenesis by accumulating in the nucleus and binding to the cullin E3 ubiquitin ligase CRL4(DCAF1) which suppresses its ubiquitination activity [69]. Merlin loss drives tumorigenesis by activating the E3 ubiquitin ligase CRL4(DCAF1), thereby inhibiting the Hippo pathway component Lats [70]. MLN4924, a NEDD8 activating enzyme (NAE) inhibitor that suppresses CRL4(DCAF1), attenuates the activation of YAP in NF2-mutant tumor cells [70]. A phase I/II clinical trial is investigating MLN4924 (Pevonedistat) alone and in combination with chemotherapy in patients with mesothelioma. MLN4924 (Pevonedistat) is a NAE inhibitor that suppresses CRL4DCAF1 and attenuates the activation of YAP in NF2-mutant tumor cells.

2.9 Cyclin-dependent kinase inhibitor 2A (CDKN2A)

Cyclin-dependent kinase inhibitor 2A is a tumor suppressor gene that is commonly mutated in MM. It encodes both proteins INK4A and ARF [71]. INK4A inhibits critical cell cycle regulators cyclin-dependent kinase 4 (CDK4) and cyclin-dependent kinase 6 (CDK6) [72]. These two kinases function to activate retinoblastoma protein (RB) and allow for cell cycle progression [72]. Without INK4A, cell cycle progression remains unchecked and allows for continuation and possible proliferation of damaged DNA. ARF acts by promoting MDM2 degradation; this degradation is necessary for the activation of p53, a widely studied tumor suppressor [73]. With p53 activated, the cell cycle is arrested and growth is suppressed. Without ARF, p53 activation is limited and cell cycle progression can continue unchecked.

Mutations in CDKN2A have been shown to be induced by environmental toxins like asbestos [74]. Furthermore, the loss of CDKN2A in MM is associated with worse prognosis and decreased survival [15, 75].

3. Multi-biomarker-driven clinical trials

The Mesothelioma Stratified Therapy Trial (MiST) is a large multi-drug phase II clinical trial evaluating the use of different biomarkers for the treatment selection in relapsed mesothelioma. BRCA1/BAP1-mutated mesothelioma treatment is being studied with Rucarapib, a PARP inhibitor. PARP enzymes are critical for cell function; they aid in DNA transcription, repair, and cell cycle regulation [76]. It is believed that by inhibiting these critical enzymes, damage will accumulate within the cell and apoptosis will be induced. In patients with absent INK4A genes, apamaciclib is being studied. Apamaciclib is a selective CDK4/6 inhibitor, theoretically working to "replace" the function of INK4A in these mutated cells to stop the cell cycle progression and tumor growth [77]. Patients with PDL1 positive mesothelioma are being treated with Atezolizumab and Bevacizumab. Atezolizumab is an anti-PDL1 antibody that selectively binds to PDL1 and prevents its interaction with B7.1 on the antigen-presenting cell (APC). This inhibits the cancer cell from utilizing PDL1 to evade the immune system [78, 79]. Lastly, for patients with no biomarkers, pembrolizumab and bemcentinib are being studied. Pembrolizumab is a monoclonal antibody against PD-1 and functions by binding PD-1 receptor on T-cells, inhibiting their binding with PDL1 [80, 81]. Bemcentinib is an AXL receptor tyrosine kinase inhibitor, a regulator of various critical cell functions including proliferation and motility, among others [82].

4. Conclusions

Over the last two decades, we have witnessed enormous efforts to identify prognostic and predictive biomarkers to inform treatment decisions in malignant mesothelioma. The medical and scientific community continue to search for optimal biomarkers to advance the field of precision medicine. Advances in molecular and diagnostic testing have not changed the current landscape of mesothelioma treatment. More biomarker-driven clinical trials are underway. The rarity of the disease makes it difficult to move these advances at a faster pace. Different pathways continue to be under investigation. These include: BAP1, NF2, CDKN2A, PD-L1, VEGF, WT-1, mesothelin, ASS, and aurora kinases. Biomarker-driven clinical trials, access to real-world data, and collaborative efforts should continue to move the field forward and help finding clinically actionable biomarkers.

Acknowledgements

There is no funding involved in this review. We would like to acknowledge the mesothelioma researchers and physicians who dedicated their career to treating mesothelioma and advance the discoveries in this field.

Conflict of interest

The authors declare no conflict of interest.

Author details

Jordyn Feinstein[1] and Muaiad Kittaneh[2]*

1 Loyola University Chicago, Maywood, USA

2 ICON, ICR, Philadelphia, USA

*Address all correspondence to: mkittaneh@me.com

References

[1] Carbone M et al. Mesothelioma: Scientific clues for prevention, diagnosis, and therapy. CA: A Cancer Journal for Clinicians. 2019;**69**(5):402-429

[2] Attanoos RL et al. Malignant mesothelioma and its non-asbestos causes. Archives of Pathology & Laboratory Medicine. 2018;**142**(6):753-760

[3] Testa JR et al. Germline BAP1 mutations predispose to malignant mesothelioma. Nature Genetics. 2011;**43**(10):1022-1025

[4] Ohta Y et al. VEGF and VEGF type C play an important role in angiogenesis and lymphangiogenesis in human malignant mesothelioma tumours. British Journal of Cancer. 1999;**81**(1):54-61

[5] Aoe K et al. Expression of vascular endothelial growth factor in malignant mesothelioma. Anticancer Research. 2006;**26**(6C):4833-4836

[6] Demirag F et al. Prognostic significance of vascular endothelial growth factor, tumor necrosis, and mitotic activity index in malignant pleural mesothelioma. Chest. 2005;**128**(5):3382-3387

[7] Zalcman G et al. Bevacizumab for newly diagnosed pleural mesothelioma in the Mesothelioma Avastin Cisplatin Pemetrexed Study (MAPS): A randomised, controlled, open-label, phase 3 trial. Lancet. 2016;**387**(10026):1405-1414

[8] Zauderer MG. A new standard for malignant pleural mesothelioma. Lancet. 2016;**387**(10026):1352-1354

[9] Dubey S et al. A phase II study of sorafenib in malignant mesothelioma: Results of Cancer and leukemia group B 30307. Journal of Thoracic Oncology. 2010;**5**(10):1655-1661

[10] Buikhuisen WA et al. A randomized phase II study adding axitinib to pemetrexed-cisplatin in patients with malignant pleural mesothelioma: A single-center trial combining clinical and translational outcomes. Journal of Thoracic Oncology. 2016;**11**(5):758-768

[11] Pagano M et al. Randomized phase II study on gemcitabine with or without ramucirumab as second-line treatment for advanced malignant pleural mesothelioma (MPM): Results of Italian Rames study. Journal of Clinical Oncology. 2020;**15**:9004

[12] Zou S et al. Arginine metabolism and deprivation in cancer therapy. Biomedicine & Pharmacotherapy. 2019;**118**:109210

[13] Fultang L et al. Molecular basis and current strategies of therapeutic arginine depletion for cancer. International Journal of Cancer. 2016;**139**(3):501-509

[14] Feun L et al. Arginine deprivation as a targeted therapy for cancer. Current Pharmaceutical Design. 2008;**14**(11):1049-1057

[15] López-Ríos F et al. Global gene expression profiling of pleural mesotheliomas: Overexpression of aurora kinases and P16/CDKN2A deletion as prognostic factors and critical evaluation of microarray-based prognostic prediction. Cancer Research. 2006;**66**(6):2970-2979

[16] Romagnoli S et al. Identification of potential therapeutic targets in malignant mesothelioma using cell-cycle gene expression analysis. The American Journal of Pathology. 2009;**174**(3):762-770

[17] Suraokar MB et al. Expression profiling stratifies mesothelioma tumors and signifies deregulation of spindle checkpoint pathway and microtubule network with therapeutic implications. Annals of Oncology. 2014;**25**(6):1184-1192

[18] Crispi S et al. Antiproliferative effect of Aurora kinase targeting in mesothelioma. Lung Cancer. 2010;**70**(3):271-279

[19] Cassandri M et al. Zinc-finger proteins in health and disease. Cell Death Discovery. 2017;**3**:17071

[20] Cedrés S et al. Expression of Wilms' tumor gene (WT1) is associated with survival in malignant pleural mesothelioma. Clinical & Translational Oncology. 2014;**16**(9):776-782

[21] Keilholz U et al. Wilms' tumour gene 1 (WT1) in human neoplasia. Leukemia. 2005;**19**(8):1318-1323

[22] Zauderer MG et al. A randomized phase II trial of adjuvant galinpepimut-S, WT-1 analogue peptide vaccine, after multimodality therapy for patients with malignant pleural mesothelioma. Clinical Cancer Research. 2017;**23**(24):7483-7489

[23] Hassan R et al. Localization of mesothelin in epithelial ovarian cancer. Applied Immunohistochemistry & Molecular Morphology. 2005;**13**(3):243-247

[24] Argani P et al. Mesothelin is overexpressed in the vast majority of ductal adenocarcinomas of the pancreas: Identification of a new pancreatic cancer marker by serial analysis of gene expression (SAGE). Clinical Cancer Research. 2001;**7**(12):3862-3868

[25] Thomas A et al. High mesothelin expression in advanced lung adenocarcinoma is associated with KRAS mutations and a poor prognosis. Oncotarget. 2015;**6**(13):11694-11703

[26] Hassan R et al. Clinical response of live-attenuated. Clinical Cancer Research. 2019;**25**(19):5787-5798

[27] Thapa B et al. Correlation of PD-L1 expression with immune cell infiltrates, genome-wide copy number aberrations and survival in mesothelioma. Journal of Clinical Oncology. 2016;**34**(15):8518-8518

[28] National Comprehensive Cancer Center Network, NCCN, Malignant Pleural Mesothelioma (Version 1.2020). Available from: https://www.nccn.org/. [Accessed: 03 September 2020]

[29] Scherpereel A et al. Nivolumab or nivolumab plus ipilimumab in patients with relapsed malignant pleural mesothelioma (IFCT-1501 MAPS2): A multicentre, open-label, randomised, non-comparative, phase 2 trial. The Lancet Oncology. 2019;**20**(2):239-253

[30] Metaxas Y et al. Pembrolizumab as palliative immunotherapy in malignant pleural mesothelioma. Journal of Thoracic Oncology. 2018;**13**(11):1784-1791

[31] Yu H et al. Tumor suppressor and deubiquitinase BAP1 promotes DNA double-strand break repair. Proceedings of the National Academy of Sciences of the United States of America. 2014;**111**(1):285-290

[32] Kittaneh M, Berkelhammer C. Detecting germline BAP1 mutations in patients with peritoneal mesothelioma: Benefits to patient and family members. Journal of Translational Medicine. 2018;**16**(1):194

[33] Bononi A et al. BAP1 regulates IP3R3-mediated Ca. Nature. 2017;**546**(7659):549-553

[34] Zhang Y et al. BAP1 links metabolic regulation of ferroptosis to tumour suppression. Nature Cell Biology. 2018;**20**(10):1181-1192

[35] Zauderer MG et al. Clinical characteristics of patients with malignant pleural mesothelioma harboring somatic BAP1 mutations. Journal of Thoracic Oncology. 2013;**8**(11):1430-1433

[36] Abdel-Rahman MH et al. Germline BAP1 mutation predisposes to uveal melanoma, lung adenocarcinoma, meningioma, and other cancers. Journal of Medical Genetics. 2011;**48**(12):856-859

[37] Carbone M et al. BAP1 cancer syndrome: Malignant mesothelioma, uveal and cutaneous melanoma, and MBAITs. Journal of Translational Medicine. 2012;**10**:179

[38] Dey A et al. Loss of the tumor suppressor BAP1 causes myeloid transformation. Science. 2012;**337**(6101):1541-1546

[39] Fan LH et al. BAP1 is a good prognostic factor in advanced non-small cell lung cancer. Clinical and Investigative Medicine. 2012;**35**(4):E182-E189

[40] Njauw CN et al. Germline BAP1 inactivation is preferentially associated with metastatic ocular melanoma and cutaneous-ocular melanoma families. PLOS One. 2012;**7**(4):e35295

[41] Wadt K et al. A cryptic BAP1 splice mutation in a family with uveal and cutaneous melanoma, and paraganglioma. Pigment Cell & Melanoma Research. 2012;**25**(6):815-818

[42] Bott M et al. The nuclear deubiquitinase BAP1 is commonly inactivated by somatic mutations and 3p21.1 losses in malignant pleural mesothelioma. Nature Genetics. 2011;**43**(7):668-672

[43] Arzt L et al. BAP1 protein is a progression factor in malignant pleural mesothelioma. Pathology Oncology Research. 2014;**20**(1):145-151

[44] Nasu M et al. High incidence of somatic BAP1 alterations in sporadic malignant mesothelioma. Journal of Thoracic Oncology. 2015;**10**(4):565-576

[45] Yoshikawa Y et al. Frequent inactivation of the BAP1 gene in epithelioid-type malignant mesothelioma. Cancer Science. 2012;**103**(5):868-874

[46] Baumann F et al. Mesothelioma patients with germline BAP1 mutations have 7-fold improved long-term survival. Carcinogenesis. 2015;**36**(1):76-81

[47] Landreville S et al. Histone deacetylase inhibitors induce growth arrest and differentiation in uveal melanoma. Clinical Cancer Research. 2012;**18**(2):408-416

[48] Kobrinski DA, Yang H, Kittaneh M. BAP1: Role in carcinogenesis and clinical implications. Translational Lung Cancer Research. 2020;**9**(Suppl 1):S60-S66

[49] Krug LM et al. Vorinostat in patients with advanced malignant pleural mesothelioma who have progressed on previous chemotherapy (VANTAGE-014): A phase 3, double-blind, randomised, placebo-controlled trial. The Lancet Oncology. 2015;**16**(4):447-456

[50] LaFave LM et al. Loss of BAP1 function leads to EZH2-dependent transformation. Nature Medicine. 2015;**21**(11):1344-1349

[51] Yamagishi M, Uchimaru K. Targeting EZH2 in cancer therapy. Current Opinion in Oncology. 2017;**29**(5):375-381

[52] Schoumacher M et al. Uveal melanoma cells are resistant to EZH2

inhibition regardless of BAP1 status. Nature Medicine. 2016;**22**(6):577-578

[53] Zauderer MG et al. Safety and efficacy of tazemetostat, an enhancer of zeste-homolog 2 inhibitor, in patients with relapsed or refractory malignant mesothelioma. Journal of Clinical Oncology. 2020;**38**(15):9058

[54] Hassan R et al. Inherited predisposition to malignant mesothelioma and overall survival following platinum chemotherapy. Proceedings of the National Academy of Sciences of the United States of America. 2019;**116**(18):9008-9013

[55] Petrilli AM, Fernández-Valle C. Role of merlin/NF2 inactivation in tumor biology. Oncogene. 2016;**35**(5):537-548

[56] Sato T, Sekido Y. NF2/merlin inactivation and potential therapeutic targets in mesothelioma. International Journal of Molecular Sciences. 2018;**19**(4):988

[57] Sekido Y et al. Neurofibromatosis type 2 (NF2) gene is somatically mutated in mesothelioma but not in lung cancer. Cancer Research. 1995;**55**(6):1227-1231

[58] Thurneysen C et al. Functional inactivation of NF2/merlin in human mesothelioma. Lung Cancer. 2009;**64**(2):140-147

[59] Bianchi AB et al. High frequency of inactivating mutations in the neurofibromatosis type 2 gene (NF2) in primary malignant mesotheliomas. Proceedings of the National Academy of Sciences of the United States of America. 1995;**92**(24):10854-10858

[60] Pan D. The hippo signaling pathway in development and cancer. Developmental Cell. 2010;**19**(4):491-505

[61] Butt Z et al. Pain and other symptoms in patients with hepatocellular carcinoma (HCC): A qualitative analysis. Journal of Clinical Oncology. 2013;**31**(15):e15187

[62] Poulikakos PI et al. Re-expression of the tumor suppressor NF2/merlin inhibits invasiveness in mesothelioma cells and negatively regulates FAK. Oncogene. 2006;**25**(44):5960-5968

[63] James MF et al. A NHERF binding site links the betaPDGFR to the cytoskeleton and regulates cell spreading and migration. Journal of Cell Science. 2004;**117**(Pt 14):2951-2961

[64] Schlaepfer DD, Mitra SK. Multiple connections link FAK to cell motility and invasion. Current Opinion in Genetics & Development. 2004;**14**(1):92-101

[65] Mitra SK, Hanson DA, Schlaepfer DD. Focal adhesion kinase: In command and control of cell motility. Nature Reviews. Molecular Cell Biology. 2005;**6**(1):56-68

[66] Fennell DA et al. Maintenance defactinib versus placebo after first-line chemotherapy in patients with merlin-stratified pleural mesothelioma: COMMAND—A double-blind, randomized, phase II study. Journal of Clinical Oncolog. 2019;**37**(10):790-798

[67] James MF et al. NF2/merlin is a novel negative regulator of mTOR complex 1, and activation of mTORC1 is associated with meningioma and schwannoma growth. Molecular and Cellular Biology. 2009;**29**(15):4250-4261

[68] López-Lago MA et al. Loss of the tumor suppressor gene NF2, encoding merlin, constitutively activates integrin-dependent mTORC1 signaling. Molecular and Cellular Biology. 2009;**29**(15):4235-4249

[69] Li W et al. Merlin/NF2 suppresses tumorigenesis by inhibiting the E3 ubiquitin ligase CRL4(DCAF1) in the nucleus. Cell. 2010;**140**(4):477-490

[70] Cooper J et al. Combined inhibition of NEDD8-activating enzyme and mTOR suppresses. Molecular Cancer Therapeutics. 2017;**16**(8):1693-1704

[71] Serrano M et al. Role of the INK4a locus in tumor suppression and cell mortality. Cell. 1996;**85**(1):27-37

[72] Serrano M, Hannon GJ, Beach D. A new regulatory motif in cell-cycle control causing specific inhibition of cyclin D/CDK4. Nature. 1993;**366**(6456):704-707

[73] Zhang Y, Xiong Y, Yarbrough WG. ARF promotes MDM2 degradation and stabilizes p53: ARF-INK4a locus deletion impairs both the Rb and p53 tumor suppression pathways. Cell. 1998;**92**(6):725-734

[74] Testa JR, Berns A. Preclinical models of malignant mesothelioma. Frontiers in Oncology. 2020;**10**:101

[75] Jennings CJ et al. Differential p16/INK4A cyclin-dependent kinase inhibitor expression correlates with chemotherapy efficacy in a cohort of 88 malignant pleural mesothelioma patients. British Journal of Cancer. 2015;**113**(1):69-75

[76] Morales J et al. Review of poly (ADP-ribose) polymerase (PARP) mechanisms of action and rationale for targeting in cancer and other diseases. Critical Reviews in Eukaryotic Gene Expression. 2014;**24**(1):15-28

[77] Sledge GW et al. MONARCH 2: Abemaciclib in combination with fulvestrant in women with HR+/HER2- advanced breast cancer who had progressed while receiving endocrine therapy. Journal of Clinical Oncology. 2017;**35**(25):2875-2884

[78] Fehrenbacher L et al. Atezolizumab versus docetaxel for patients with previously treated non-small-cell lung cancer (POPLAR): A multicentre, open-label, phase 2 randomised controlled trial. Lancet. 2016;**387**(10030):1837-1846

[79] Rosenberg JE et al. Atezolizumab in patients with locally advanced and metastatic urothelial carcinoma who have progressed following treatment with platinum-based chemotherapy: A single-arm, multicentre, phase 2 trial. Lancet. 2016;**387**(10031):1909-1920

[80] Robert C et al. Anti-programmed-death-receptor-1 treatment with pembrolizumab in ipilimumab-refractory advanced melanoma: A randomised dose-comparison cohort of a phase 1 trial. Lancet. 2014;**384**(9948):1109-1117

[81] Hamid O et al. Safety and tumor responses with lambrolizumab (anti-PD-1) in melanoma. The New England Journal of Medicine. 2013;**369**(2):134-144

[82] Zhu C, Wei Y, Wei X. AXL receptor tyrosine kinase as a promising anti-cancer approach: Functions, molecular mechanisms and clinical applications. Molecular Cancer. 2019;**18**(1):153

Chapter 7

Genetic Alterations of Malignant Pleural Mesothelima

Benjamin Wadowski, David T. Severson, Raphael Bueno and Assunta De Rienzo

Abstract

Malignant pleural mesothelioma (MPM) is a highly aggressive tumor that arises from the mesothelial cells lining the pleural cavity. Asbestos is considered the major factor in the pathogenesis of this malignancy, with more than 80% of patients with a history of asbestos exposure. MPM is characterized by a long latency period, typically 20–40 years from the time of asbestos exposure to diagnosis, suggesting that multiple somatic genetic alterations are required for the tumorigenic conversion of a mesothelial cell. In the last few years, advancements in next-generation sequencing and "–omics" technologies have revolutionized the field of genomics and medical diagnosis. The focus of this chapter is to summarize recent studies which explore the molecular mechanisms underlying this disease and identify potential therapeutic targets in MPM.

Keywords: pleural mesothelioma, next-generation sequencing, transcriptome, exome sequencing, tumor suppressor gene

1. Introduction

Malignant pleural mesothelioma (MPM) is a lethal cancer of the mesothelial cells lining the pleural cavity and, less frequently, the pericardium, peritoneum, and tunica vaginalis [1]. Many years after the peak of asbestos use in United States, 3200 cases of MPM continue to be diagnosed annually, indicating that the U.S. population remains at risk of exposure to asbestos and development of mesothelioma [2]. There are two major histological variants: epithelioid, which accounts for about 60% of cases and has the more favorable prognosis, and sarcomatoid, whose incidence is 10%. The remaining cases demonstrate histologic characteristics of both types and are classified as biphasic [3]. The prognosis for patients with MPM is poor, with a median survival of 5–15 months [3]. However, some patients with early MPM who undergo multimodality therapy including surgical resection and chemotherapy demonstrate longer-term survival of up to 25% at 5 years [4].

Many studies have shown a causal relationship between exposure to asbestos and mesothelioma (reviewed by Bianche et al. [5]). Although it has been suggested that brief asbestos exposure is sufficient to induce disease, MPM is the consequence of prolonged exposure in most cases. However, only a small percentage of individuals exposed to asbestos develop MPM, suggesting that genetic predisposition may modulate the effect of exposure to asbestos. In addition, 20% of MPM cases with unknown asbestos exposure have been related to other risk factors such as radiation therapy and thorotrast [6].

Studies conducted on large numbers of patients indicate that the time between asbestos exposure and diagnosis of MPM is generally more than 20 years. The molecular mechanisms for the transformation of mesothelial cells are unknown; it has been suggested that asbestos induces multiple chromosomal aberrations, particularly deletions, facilitating oncogenesis [7].

Investigations prior to the advent of next-generation sequencing (NGS) revealed the complexity of the genetic alterations observed in MPM tumors by using karyotypic and comparative genomic hybridization (CGH) analyses [8, 9]. Chromosomal losses were found to be more frequent than gains and particular chromosomal regions (1p22, 3p21, 4q, 6q, 9p21, 13q13–14, 15q11–15, and 22q12) were deleted at higher frequency in MPM tissues and cell lines [10–12]. Two tumor suppressor genes (TSGs) were identified by positional cloning approaches: *CDKN2A* at 9p21 and *NF2* at 22q12. In the last few years, the genetic landscape of MPM has been characterized using high-throughput technologies [13–15]. The focus of this chapter is to summarize the major genetic changes occurring in MPM as identified by high-throughput sequencing and to describe the novel insights obtained through transcriptomic studies.

2. Exome sequencing studies

NGS technologies have allowed the sequencing of DNA and RNA at unprecedented speed, uncovering potential driver genes and creating novel biological applications [16]. In the last decade, NGS has been used to detect driver genetic mutations in cancer and provide new insights into tumorigenesis.

Shotgun pyrosequencing was used to characterize RNA expression levels and mutations of four patients in the first effort to investigate MPM by NGS. Several different mutations were found in the four transcriptomes. In addition, RNA editing gene deletions and gene silencing were identified [17].

In 2010, the first whole genome sequence of one MPM tumor and matching normal tissue was conducted using a combination of sequencing-by-synthesis and pyrosequencing methodologies [18]. This study showed that aneuploidy and chromosomal rearrangements were more numerous than point mutations in this tumor. One large deletion in the dipeptidyl peptidase like 10 (*DPP10*) gene, altering the expression of the corresponding transcript, was further investigated in 53 additional MPM tumors. Patients expressing *DPP10* had statistically longer survival compared to patients lacking *DPP10* expression [18].

In 2016, Bueno et al. conducted an extensive analysis of the mutational landscape of MPM. Ninety-nine MPM tumors were examined by whole exome sequencing, whereas additional 103 samples were characterized by targeted exome sequencing [13]. *BAP1*, *NF2*, *TP53*, *SETD2*, *DDX3X*, *ULK2*, *RYR2*, *CFAP45*, *SETDB1* and *DDX51* were found to be significantly mutated (q-score ≥ 0.8), and recurrent mutations were found in *SF3B1* (2%) and *TRAF7* (2%).

In 2018, The Cancer Genome Atlas (TCGA) program performed a comprehensive molecular profiling of 74 primary MPM samples including exome sequencing, copy-number arrays, mRNA sequencing, noncoding RNA profiling, DNA methylation, and reverse-phase protein arrays [15]. The significantly mutated genes in this study were *BAP1*, *NF2*, *TP53*, *LATS2*, and *SETD2*. Furthermore, this study identified a new near-haploid molecular MPM subtype.

The TCGA study performed a comparison of the significantly mutated genes between the Bueno and TCGA cohorts [15]. This analysis identified five genes that were frequently mutated in both studies: BRCA1-associated protein-1 (*BAP1*), neurofibromin 2 (*NF2*), tumor protein P53 (*TP53*), SET domain containing 2, histone lysine methyltransferase (*SETD2*), and SET domain bifurcated histone lysine methyltransferase 1 (*SETDB1*). The large tumor suppressor kinase 2 (*LATS2*) gene was found frequently altered in the TCGA cohort alone, whereas four additional genes, DEAD-box helicase 3 X-linked (*DDX3X*), Unc-51-like autophagy-activating kinase 2 (*ULK2*), ryanodine receptor 2 (*RYR2*), and DEAD-box helicase 51 (*DDX51*) were identified as commonly mutated in the series from Bueno et al. (**Table 1**).

2.1 BAP1

BAP1 is located on the short (p) arm of chromosome 3, at position 21.1., a region frequently deleted in MPM [9]. This gene encodes for a deubiquitinase involved in cell cycle regulation, modulation of gene transcription, cellular differentiation, and DNA repair [19]. *BAP1* is one of the most commonly mutated genes in MPM [13, 15, 20, 21]. Germline *BAP1* mutations have been linked to the development of *BAP1* tumor predisposition syndrome, which includes uveal and cutaneous melanoma, atypical Spitz tumors, renal cell carcinoma, and MPM. In all these malignancies but MPM, *BAP1* mutations are associated with poor prognosis [22, 23]. In contrast, some studies have shown that patients with MPM carrying *BAP1* mutations have longer overall survival compared to patients with wild-type *BAP1* [24, 25]. In one study, BAP1 immunohistochemistry (IHC) was performed using tissue microarray including 229 MPM tumors. The results showed that loss of BAP1 nuclear staining was associated with longer median survival of 16.11 months (95% CI: 12.16–20.06) versus 6.34 months for patients with nuclear BAP1 staining (95% CI: 5.34–7.34) ($P < 0.01$) [24]. Baumann et al. compared the survival in 23 patients with MPM carrying germline mutations in *BAP1* with a control group of MPM patients from the Surveillance, Epidemiology, and End Results (SEER) database and found a 7-fold increase in long-term survival in patients with BAP1 mutation [25].

Given its prevalence in MPM, loss of nuclear BAP1 expression by IHC is commonly used as a diagnostic marker in MPM [26, 27].

Recently, *BAP1* status has been associated with drug response [28, 29]. *In vitro* studies showed MPM cell lines carrying *BAP1* mutations were significantly less sensitive to gemcitabine compared to wild-type cells. Silencing of *BAP1* in MPM

Gene symbol	Gene ID	Chromosomal location	Number of mutations in Bueno's cohort	Number of mutations in Hmeljak's cohort	Total
BAP1	ENSG00000163930	3p21.1	55	17	72
NF2	ENSG00000186575	22q12.2	39	19	58
TP53	ENSG00000141510	17p31.1	17	10	27
SETD2	ENSG00000181555	3p21.31	18	8	26
SETDB1	ENSG00000143379	1q21	7	3	10
LATS2	ENSG00000150457	13q12.11	2	9	11
DDX3X	ENSG00000215301	Xp11.4	8	0	8
RYR2	ENSG00000198626	1q43	4	1	5
ULK2	ENSG00000083290	17p11.2	4	0	4
DDX51	ENSG00000185163	12q24.33	3	0	3
Total			157	67	224

Table 1.
Number of mutations in each gene in the two studies.

wild-type cells significantly increased resistance to gemcitabine, suggesting a role of *BAP1* in drug response [28]. Kumar et al. performed a retrospective study analyzing presence or absence of nuclear BAP1 by IHC in MPM tumors from 60 patients in the MS01 trial (NCT00075699) [29]. Nuclear BAP1 expression was associated with a small but statistically nonsignificant decrease in survival in patients treated with vinorelbine.

2.2 NF2

NF2 is located on the long (q) arm of chromosome 22 at position 12.2. Loss of chromosome 22 is a common alteration in MPM [9]. This gene codes for a protein known as merlin (moesinezrin-radixin-like protein) or schwannomin, which regulates key signaling pathways involved in cell growth, adhesion, and microtubule stabilization [30]. Germline mutation or chromosomal deletion of *NF2* causes the neurofibromatosis type 2 syndrome, which is associated with tumors of the cranial and peripheral nerves as well as meningioma and ependymoma [31]. Germline mutations in *NF2* have also been linked to MPM; however, patients with both neurofibromatosis type 2 syndrome and MPM are extremely rare [32]. Recent studies have shown that *NF2* mutations occur in 14–19% of MPM [13–15, 20]. In addition, karyotype and/or FISH analyses demonstrated that 56% MPMs have shown loss of chromosome 22q. Deletions of 22q are more frequently associated with epithelioid than non-epithelioid MPM ($p = 0.037$) [20].

In 2009, a study suggested that *NF2* may be inactivated by upstream regulators in MPM tumors where no *NF2* aberration can be detected [33]. In an investigation of 204 MPM patients, low cytoplasmic merlin expression was found to predict shorter recurrence interval and shorter overall survival [34]. Lopez-Lago et al. investigated the association between loss of merlin and mTORC1 activation in MPM cell lines and found that merlin-negative or merlin-depleted cell lines were more sensitive to the growth-inhibitory effect of rapamycin [35]. In 2014, low merlin expression was found to be associated to increased sensitivity of MPM cell lines to a FAK inhibitor, VS-471 [36]. However, in clinical trials, the FAK inhibitor defactinib did not improve progression free or overall survival in patients with MPM after first-line chemotherapy [37].

2.3 TP53

Located at 17p31.1, *TP53* codes for tumor protein p53 (p53), which is a sequence-specific DNA binding protein that regulates transcription and has a tumor suppressor function controlling cell apoptosis in presence of DNA damage [38]. Named "the guardian of the genome," p53 is involved in many cellular processes such as checkpoint control, cellular senescence, and BCL-2 mediated apoptosis [39]. *TP53* is, overall, the most frequently altered gene in human cancer [40]. The frequency of *TP53* mutations in MPM across different studies is variable, but overall it is much lower than in other solid tumors [13–15, 20]. *TP53* was significantly more frequently mutated in women (10/40; 25%) compared to men (17/169, 10%) (Fisher's exact $P = 0.044$) when all samples included in two large MPM studies [13, 15] were analyzed. In addition, Bueno et al. reported that MPM patients with mutations in *TP53* had shorter overall survival than those with wild-type *TP53* ($p = 0.0167$) [13].

2.4 SETD2

SETD2 maps to 3p21.31. It encodes a histone methyltransferase specific for lysine-36 of histone H3 which regulates transcription through epigenetic mechanisms [41]. Inactivating *SETD2* mutations have been identified in multiple cancers [42]. In particular, targeted sequencing revealed *SETD2* bi-allelic inactivation in clear cell renal cell carcinoma tumors suggesting for the first time that *SETD2* may contribute to tumor formation [43]. In MPM, single nucleotide mutations in *SETD2* as well as 3p losses are frequently observed [13, 15, 44]. In the last few years, *SETD2* alterations have been linked to mechanisms of resistance to DNA-damaging chemotherapy in several cancers [45, 46].

2.5 SETDB1

SETDB1 is positioned at 1q21, another region frequently deleted in MPM [9], and codes for histone-lysine N-methyltransferase *SETDB1* which trimethylates Lys-9 of histone H3 [47]. As an epigenetic modulator, *SETDB1* has a critical role in several biological processes such as embryonic development, adipocyte differentiation, and inflammation, as well as providing regulation of several signaling pathways including the P13K-AKT axis, p53, the STAT1-CCND1/CDK6 axis, and gene promoter methylation [48].

Targeted deep sequencing has revealed somatic *SETDB1* mutations in 10% (7/69) patients with MPM [49]. No significant correlation between mutation in *SETDB1* and survival was found ($p = 0.351$). Mutations in *SETDB1* were also identified in 3% (7/202) of MPMs in a different cohort [13]. Hmeljak et al. found that *SETDB1* mutations were present together with *TP53* and extensive loss of heterozygosity in 3% of MPM. This rare genomic subtype was associated with female sex and younger age at diagnosis [15].

2.6 LATS2

LATS2, located on 13q12.11, encodes for a serine/threonine kinase which is involved in a broad array of programs such as cell cycle regulation, cell motility, and differentiation [50]. Loss of *LATS2*, either through copy number alteration or mutation, has been identified in several different cancer types [51], as well as in MPM [15, 52]. In a cohort of 266 MPM samples, mutations in *LATS2* were observed in 5% of the samples, with lower frequency in epithelioid compared to non-epithelioid samples. In addition, *LATS2* mutations were more frequent in patients without asbestos exposure (7%) than those exposed (2%) [53]. Another study identified a new molecular subgroup of MPM characterized by a co-occurring mutation in *LATS2* and *NF2*. MPM patients in this subgroup had poor prognosis compared to the cohort at large [54].

Several investigations have linked *LATS2* to the transcription regulator YAP involved in the Hippo pathways. Mizuno et al. found that inactivation of *LATS2* leads to YAP overexpression, which, when knocked down, inhibits cell motility and invasion *in vitro* [55]. Another study demonstrated that *LATS2* is a key binding partner of AJUBA, which suppresses YAP activity in mesothelioma [56].

2.7 DDX3X

DDX3X resides on Xp11.4 and encodes an ATP-dependent RNA helicase with RNA-independent ATPase activity stimulated by either DNA or RNA [57]. DDX3X has both cytoplasmic and nuclear functions including translation, regulation of transcription, pre-mRNA splicing, and mRNA export [58]. Its functions are complex and varied: *DDX3X* has been recognized as both an oncogene and a tumor suppressor, sometimes within the context of a single type of cancer [59]. An analysis of the COSMIC database found that 12% of genetic abnormalities in *DDX3* are typical for tumor suppressors, while 81% are more typical for gain of function [59].

2.8 RYR2

RYR2 is located at 1q43. It encodes a member of the ryanodine receptor family of calcium channels, highly expressed in cardiac muscle but also found in smooth muscle and the nervous system [60]. The release of calcium from the sarcoplasmic reticulum into the cytoplasm via RyR2 triggers contraction in myocytes, whereas in the brain, it aids in functions related to learning and memory [60]. Although mutations in *RYR2* have been reported in other cancers [61], *RYR2* mutations in MPM have been identified only in one study [13].

2.9 ULK2

ULK2 maps on 17p11.2. It codes for an Atg1 homolog and serine/threonine kinase which normally localizes to the membrane of autophagosomes and plays a key role in autophagy, particularly in the setting of nutrient deprivation or mTOR inhibition [62]. *ULK2* has been linked to the development of astrocytoma [63], and colorectal cancer [64]. Rare *ULK2* mutations have been identified in MPM [13]. In spheroid models of MPM, autophagy was successfully inhibited by the ULK1/2 inhibitor MRT 68921 [65].

2.10 DDX51

DDX51 resides on 12q24.33. It is a ribosome synthesis factor required for the formation of the 3′ end of 28S rRNA [66]. Abnormal function of *DDX51* has been linked to NSCLC, leukemia, and breast cancer [67–69]. Few *DDX51* mutations have been found in MPM [13].

3. Transcriptome sequencing studies

Since gene expression is linked to tumor behavior, bulk expression profiling of tumors has revolutionized our understanding of cancer by giving insight into the expression levels of thousands of genes measured at once. In addition, the allocation of cancer specimens into molecular clusters having similar biological and clinical characteristics has improved the understanding of the molecular biology of tumors and identified both actionable targets for therapies as well as biomarkers for prediction of response [70].

In 2005, Gordon et al. profiled 40 MPM tumors using microarray technologies [71]. Four normal pleura specimens and four normal lung tissues were included in the analysis as controls because MPM arises from mesothelial cells of the pleura and often involves the lung parenchyma [71]. Unsupervised cluster analysis revealed four distinct subclasses with two, named C1 and C2, consisting only of MPM samples. These two clusters had epithelial (88%) and mixed (78%) subtypes, respectively, showing a partial correlation with tumor histology. Differential gene expression analysis demonstrated genes related to cytoskeletal/support, such as keratins, cadherins, and other proteoglycans, were over-expressed in cluster C1, whereas genes associated with extracellular matrix and structural proteins such as collagen, actin, biglycan, and fibronectin were highly expressed in subclass C2 [71].

In 2014, a study from de Reynies et al. generated a transcriptomic classification of MPM using 38 primary cultures [72]. Consensus clustering of the expression profiles identified two groups of MPM, C1 and C2, which are partially related to histology. Epithelioid MPM were found in both clusters, whereas sarcomatoid tumors clustered only in C2. In addition, tumor samples in C1 tended to have more frequent mutations in *BAP1* ($P = 0.09$) and deletions of the chromosomal region 3p21 ($P < 0.01$), where *BAP1* is located. Furthermore, 40 genes that discriminated the two groups were used to validate the molecular classification in 108 MPM tumors. Survival analyses showed that patients in C2 had shorter survival compared to the survival of patients in cluster C1 ($P = 0.02$). This difference persisted when only epithelioid samples were included ($P < 0.01$) [72]. Pathway analyses revealed that the most deregulated pathways were those related to the epithelial-to-mesenchymal transition (EMT) process [72].

In 2016, a seminal publication on genomics in MPM described unsupervised consensus clustering of RNA sequencing data from 211 MPM tumors. This analysis classified the samples into four distinct molecular clusters: epithelioid, biphasic-epithelioid (biphasic-E), biphasic-sarcomatoid (biphasic-S), and sarcomatoid [13]. The clusters were loosely associated with the spectrum from epithelioid to sarcomatoid histology. Epithelioid and biphasic samples were distributed in all four subgroups, whereas sarcomatoid tumors were only in one cluster. Biphasic samples clustered according to the proportion of epithelioid and sarcomatoid cells contained in the specimen; biphasic tumors with the highest portion of sarcomatoid cells grouped with the sarcomatoid samples. Notably, patients in the epithelioid cluster had longer overall survival compared to the survival of patients in the other three groups. Differential expression analysis of the sarcomatoid and epithelioid clusters revealed that genes related to the EMT process were differently expressed between the two groups, and that ratio of two genes *CLDN15* and *VIM* (C/V score) significantly differentiated the four clusters [13].

A different approach to classify MPM tumors was used by Hmeljak et al. [15]. To determine whether a multi-platform molecular profiling may offer additional power to identify subsets of MPM, two clustering algorithms, iCluster [73] and PARADIGM [74] were used to integrate somatic copy-number alteration, gene expression, and epigenetic data from 74 MPM samples. Both algorithms grouped the samples into four distinct clusters with high concordance between the two methods in the assignment of the sample into the groups. Survival analyses showed significant differences in survival across the four groups. In addition, the four clusters were significantly associated with histology: cluster 1 contained many epithelioid samples, whereas cluster 4 was enriched for sarcomatoid tumors as found in previous studies [13, 71, 72]. This study, using a small number of samples, mostly epithelial, confirmed that genes related to the EMT process were differentially expressed between the two most extreme clusters [15].

In 2019, unsupervised clustering of microarray profiles assigned 63 primary MPMs into four groups (C1A, C1B, C2A, and C2B) [75]. Then, a meta-analysis of mesothelioma expression profiles was conducted to compare these clusters with the groups from previous classifications [13, 15, 71, 72, 75, 76]. This analysis identified two highly correlated MPM clusters present in all expression profiles, which corresponded to the extreme epithelioid and the sarcomatoid phenotypes. The remaining groups did not associate closely suggesting that they may represent different points of a continuum or "histo-molecular gradient" of epithelioid and sarcomatoid components. A deconvolution approach was used to identify novel insights into the intra-tumor heterogeneity of MPM by dissecting whole tissue RNA-sequencing signatures into biologically relevant components. This analysis produced two molecular signatures of 150 genes, E-score and S-score, which were related to histology and recapitulated the molecular classification. These signatures reflected the proportion of epithelioid-like and sarcomatoid-like components within each MPM tumor. In addition, the proportions of these cellular components were significantly associated with prognosis [75].

Regardless of the metric used, the whole transcriptome studies indicate that MPM is characterized by a molecular gradient associated with the EMT process. Most recently, the relationship between the C/V score [18] and other published metrics [75, 77] associated with the EMT process has been investigated [78] demonstrating a significant correlation of the C/V score with other molecular signatures. These results indicate that the ratio of just two genes can be sufficient to determine the "EMT-component" in each MPM [78].

4. Clinical significance

While further work is needed before these data can be applied directly to patient care, an understanding of the molecular heterogeneity of MPM and the mutations that contribute to different subtypes can have a meaningful impact on the direction of clinical research in this field. In 2014, *in vitro* and tumor xenograft experiments suggested that low Merlin (NF2 protein) expression may predict increased sensitivity of MPM cells to a FAK inhibitor, VS-4718 [36]. Subsequently, the use of defactinib, a FAK inhibitor, was investigated in the neoadjuvant setting for surgically resectable disease (a "window of opportunity" study). The treatment was well tolerated and resulted in successful inhibition of FAK, as well as inhibition of multiple cancer stem cell markers such as CD133 and SOX2 (Bueno et al., 2018 personal communication, International Mesothelioma Interest Group (IMIG) Conference, 2016 Birmingham UK). The use of defactinib as maintenance therapy following first-line chemotherapy in advanced MPM was also assessed in the COMMAND trial, a phase II randomized placebo-controlled study. Three hundred forty-four patients were stratified by merlin expression and randomized; however, there was no significant improvement in progression-free survival (4.1 [95% CI: 2.9–5.6] versus 4 [95% CI: 2.9–4.2] months) or overall survival (12.7 [95% CI: 9.1–21] versus 13.6 [95% CI: 9.6 to 21.2] months) of patients treated with defactinib compared to placebo [37].

Knowledge of key mutations in MPM has guided investigations into other forms of targeted therapy, although many are still at the preclinical stage. For example, LaFave and colleagues found evidence that loss of Bap1 expression increases Ezh2 expression in xenograft and *Bap1* knock-out mice and enhances sensitivity to EZH2 inhibition *in vitro*. Szlosarek and colleagues studied arginine deprivation in 68 patients with advanced ASS1-deficient malignant pleural mesothelioma (defined by $>50\%$ low expressor cells on immunohistochemical analysis) [79]. Treatment with the deprivation agent ADI-PEG20 improved progression-free survival (3.2 vs. 2 months, $p = 0.03$) with no significant difference in life expectancy or adverse events.

Beyond identifying therapeutic targets, multi-omic data have enhanced the understanding of tumor biology, providing novel ways to stratify patients, determining prognosis and predicting sensitivity to existing treatments (reviewed in [80]).

We have developed a gene expression ratio-based method to translate expression profiling data into clinical tests based on the expression levels of a small number of genes [81]. This method uses standard supervised methods for microarray analysis to compare gene expression in two types of tissues differing by a single clinical parameter such as histology or outcome. Genes with the most significant difference in expression are selected and used in combination to calculate ratios of gene expression able to predict the clinical parameter associated with a random patient sample.

Using this method, a 6-gene 3-ratio test has been developed to distinguish MPM from adenocarcinoma using resection specimens and fine needle biopsies [81, 82]. A similar approach was used to generate a 4-gene 3-ratio prognostic test to identify patients likely to benefit from tumor resection in the preoperative setting [83, 84], as well as a 4-gene 3-ratio signature to distinguish the epithelioid from the sarcomatoid MPM subtype [85].

Despite rapidly decreasing sequencing costs [86], there remain several barriers to introducing the use of NGS technology in clinical practice, especially in MPM. In many solid tumors, the development of targeted sequencing panels has led to targeted therapies and prediction of survival of cancer patients. MPM is rare, making large-scale validation studies difficult to perform, and heterogeneous, characterized by mutations highly variable among tumors. In addition, loss of TSGs is a common feature of MPM making potential treatments associated with these genes difficult to be applied to real life treatment. Clinical trials focused on specific mutated genes [29, 37] have been infrequent and the results never translated to practice. Transcriptome analyses have classified MPM patients into several groups stratifying patients into categories of risk; however, a substantial margin of error in these predictions persists because the sensitivity and specificity of these tests are difficult to define [87]. Precision medicine based on cancer genomics is still far from being applied in clinical practice in MPM. Nevertheless, we are confident in the value of NGS for personalized medicine and believe additional efforts are needed for the implementation of NGS in identifying patients who might benefit from targeted treatments.

5. Conclusions

NGS has revolutionized the study of human genetics by transforming our ability to analyze the causes of disease, develop new diagnostics, and identify potential therapeutic targets. NGS studies have led to the discovery of several commonly mutated genes in MPM [13, 15]. Although analyses of transcriptome data have contributed to the understanding of the molecular biology of MPM subtypes, these studies were based on bulk profiling where tumors were profiled as a single entity averaging the gene expression of all the cells in the specimen and ignoring the intra-tumor heterogeneity that regulates many critical aspects of tumor biology [88]. The importance of intra-tumor heterogeneity in MPM is becoming evident. Future single-cell RNA sequencing work will be able to elucidate molecular roles of immune infiltrates and stroma in MPM as well as to clarify whether the molecular mechanisms associated with the genetic heterogeneity are due to subclonal mutations, epigenetic programs, or other environmental factors such as cell-cell interaction or nutrient availability.

Acknowledgements

This work was supported by grants to RB from the National Cancer Institute (NCI 2 R01 CA120528-11A1) and the International Mesothelioma Program at Brigham and Women's Hospital. The study sponsors played no role in the study design, collection, analysis, interpretation of data, writing of the report, or decision to submit the chapter for publication.

Conflict of interest

The authors disclose no potential conflicts of interest. Dr. Bueno reports grants from Medgenome, grants from Roche, grants from Verastem, grants from Merck, grants from Gristone, grants from Epizyme, grants from Siemens, grants from

NCI, grants from DoD, and grants from NIH. In addition, Dr. Bueno has a patent 7,622,260 licensed to BWH, a patent 8,450,057 licensed to BWH, a patent 8,551,700 licensed to BWH, and a patent 9,446,050 licensed to BWH, and Patents/Equity in Navigation Sciences.

Author details

Benjamin Wadowski, David T. Severson, Raphael Bueno and Assunta De Rienzo*
The Thoracic Surgery Oncology Laboratory and the International Mesothelioma Program, Division of Thoracic Surgery and the Lung Center, Brigham and Women's Hospital and Harvard Medical School, Boston, MA, USA

*Address all correspondence to: aderienzo@bwh.harvard.edu

References

[1] Robinson BW, Lake RA. Advances in malignant mesothelioma. The New England Journal of Medicine. 2005;**353**(15):1591-1603

[2] Henley SJ, Larson TC, Wu M, et al. Mesothelioma incidence in 50 states and the District of Columbia, United States, 2003-2008. International Journal of Occupational and Environmental Health. 2013;**19**(1):1-10

[3] Raja S, Murthy SC, Mason DP. Malignant pleural mesothelioma. Current Oncology Reports. 2011;**13**(4):259-264

[4] Sugarbaker DJ, Wolf AS, Chirieac LR, et al. Clinical and pathological features of three-year survivors of malignant pleural mesothelioma following extrapleural pneumonectomy. European Journal of Cardio-Thoracic Surgery. 2011;**40**(2):298-303

[5] Bianchi C, Bianchi T. Malignant mesothelioma: Global incidence and relationship with asbestos. Industrial Health. 2007;**45**(3):379-387

[6] Prazakova S, Thomas PS, Sandrini A, Yates DH. Asbestos and the lung in the 21st century: An update. The Clinical Respiratory Journal. 2014;**8**(1):1-10

[7] Mutsaers SE. The mesothelial cell. The International Journal of Biochemistry & Cell Biology. 2004;**36**(1):9-16

[8] Carbone M, Kratzke RA, Testa JR. The pathogenesis of mesothelioma. Seminars in Oncology. 2002;**29**(1):2-17

[9] Lee WC, Testa JR. Somatic genetic alterations in human malignant mesothelioma (review). International Journal of Oncology. 1999;**14**(1):181-188

[10] Balsara BR, Bell DW, Sonoda G, et al. Comparative genomic hybridization and loss of heterozygosity analyses identify a common region of deletion at 15q11.1-15 in human malignant mesothelioma. Cancer Research. 1999;**59**(2):450-454

[11] De Rienzo A, Balsara BR, Apostolou S, Jhanwar SC, Testa JR. Loss of heterozygosity analysis defines a 3-cM region of 15q commonly deleted in human malignant mesothelioma. Oncogene. 2001;**20**(43):6245-6249

[12] De Rienzo A, Jhanwar SC, Testa JR. Loss of heterozygosity analysis of 13q and 14q in human malignant mesothelioma. Genes, Chromosomes & Cancer. 2000;**28**(3):337-341

[13] Bueno R, Stawiski EW, Goldstein LD, et al. Comprehensive genomic analysis of malignant pleural mesothelioma identifies recurrent mutations, gene fusions and splicing alterations. Nature Genetics. 2016;**48**(4):407-416

[14] Guo G, Chmielecki J, Goparaju C, et al. Whole-exome sequencing reveals frequent genetic alterations in *BAP1*, *NF2*, *CDKN2A*, and CUL1 in malignant pleural mesothelioma. Cancer Research. 2015;**75**(2):264-269

[15] Hmeljak J, Sanchez-Vega F, Hoadley KA, et al. Integrative molecular characterization of malignant pleural mesothelioma. Cancer Discovery. 2018;**8**(12):1548-1565

[16] Zhang J, Chiodini R, Badr A, Zhang G. The impact of next-generation sequencing on genomics. Journal of Genetics and Genomics. 2011;**38**(3):95-109

[17] Sugarbaker DJ, Richards WG, Gordon GJ, et al. Transcriptome sequencing of malignant pleural mesothelioma tumors. Proceedings of the National Academy of Sciences of the United States of America. 2008;**105**(9):3521-3526

[18] Bueno R, De Rienzo A, Dong L, et al. Second generation sequencing of the mesothelioma tumor genome. PLoS One. 2010;**5**(5):e10612

[19] Carbone M, Yang H, Pass HI, Krausz T, Testa JR, Gaudino G. BAP1 and cancer. Nature Reviews. Cancer. 2013;**13**(3):153-159

[20] De Rienzo A, Archer MA, Yeap BY, et al. Gender-specific molecular and clinical features underlie malignant pleural mesothelioma. Cancer Research. 2016;**76**(2):319-328

[21] Nasu M, Emi M, Pastorino S, et al. High incidence of somatic BAP1 alterations in sporadic malignant mesothelioma. Journal of Thoracic Oncology. 2015;**10**(4):565-576

[22] Rai K, Pilarski R, Cebulla CM, Abdel-Rahman MH. Comprehensive review of BAP1 tumor predisposition syndrome with report of two new cases. Clinical Genetics. 2016;**89**(3):285-294

[23] Wang A, Papneja A, Hyrcza M, Al-Habeeb A, Ghazarian D. Gene of the month: BAP1. Journal of Clinical Pathology. 2016;**69**(9):750-753

[24] Farzin M, Toon CW, Clarkson A, et al. Loss of expression of BAP1 predicts longer survival in mesothelioma. Pathology. 2015;**47**(4):302-307

[25] Baumann F, Flores E, Napolitano A, et al. Mesothelioma patients with germline BAP1 mutations have 7-fold improved long-term survival. Carcinogenesis. 2015;**36**(1):76-81

[26] Carbone M, Adusumilli PS, Alexander HR Jr, et al. Mesothelioma: Scientific clues for prevention, diagnosis, and therapy. CA: A Cancer Journal for Clinicians. 2019;**69**(5):402-429

[27] Pillappa R, Maleszewski JJ, Sukov WR, et al. Loss of BAP1 expression in atypical mesothelial proliferations helps to predict malignant mesothelioma. The American Journal of Surgical Pathology. 2018;**42**(2):256-263

[28] Guazzelli A, Meysami P, Bakker E, et al. BAP1 status determines the sensitivity of malignant mesothelioma cells to gemcitabine treatment. International Journal of Molecular Sciences. 2019;**20**(2):429

[29] Kumar N, Alrifai D, Kolluri KK, et al. Retrospective response analysis of BAP1 expression to predict the clinical activity of systemic cytotoxic chemotherapy in mesothelioma. Lung Cancer. 2019;**127**:164-166

[30] Smole Z, Thoma CR, Applegate KT, et al. Tumor suppressor NF2/merlin is a microtubule stabilizer. Cancer Research. 2014;**74**(1):353-362

[31] Petrilli AM, Fernandez-Valle C. Role of merlin/NF2 inactivation in tumor biology. Oncogene. 2016;**35**(5):537-548

[32] Baser ME, De Rienzo A, Altomare D, et al. Neurofibromatosis 2 and malignant mesothelioma. Neurology. 2002;**59**(2):290-291

[33] Thurneysen C, Opitz I, Kurtz S, Weder W, Stahel RA, Felley-Bosco E. Functional inactivation of NF2/merlin in human mesothelioma. Lung Cancer. 2009;**64**(2):140-147

[34] Meerang M, Berard K, Friess M, et al. Low merlin expression and high Survivin labeling index are indicators for poor prognosis in patients with malignant pleural mesothelioma. Molecular Oncology. 2016;**10**(8):1255-1265

[35] Lopez-Lago MA, Okada T, Murillo MM, Socci N, Giancotti FG. Loss of the tumor suppressor gene NF2, encoding merlin, constitutively activates integrin-dependent mTORC1 signaling. Molecular and Cellular Biology. 2009;**29**(15):4235-4249

[36] Shapiro IM, Kolev VN, Vidal CM, et al. Merlin deficiency predicts FAK inhibitor sensitivity: A synthetic lethal relationship. Science Translational Medicine. 2014;**6**(237):237ra268

[37] Fennell DA, Baas P, Taylor P, et al. Maintenance defactinib versus placebo after first-line chemotherapy in patients with merlin-stratified pleural mesothelioma: COMMAND-A double-blind, randomized, phase II study. Journal of Clinical Oncology. 2019;**37**(10):790-798

[38] Laptenko O, Prives C. Transcriptional regulation by p53: One protein, many possibilities. Cell Death and Differentiation. 2006;**13**(6):951-961

[39] Anbarasan T, Bourdon JC. The emerging landscape of p53 isoforms in physiology, cancer and degenerative diseases. International Journal of Molecular Sciences. 2019;**20**(24):6257

[40] Kandoth C, McLellan MD, Vandin F, et al. Mutational landscape and significance across 12 major cancer types. Nature. 2013;**502**(7471):333-339

[41] Yuan W, Xie J, Long C, et al. Heterogeneous nuclear ribonucleoprotein L is a subunit of human KMT3a/Set2 complex required for H3 Lys-36 trimethylation activity in vivo. The Journal of Biological Chemistry. 2009;**284**(23):15701-15707

[42] Li J, Duns G, Westers H, Sijmons R, van den Berg A, Kok K. *SETD2*: An epigenetic modifier with tumor suppressor functionality. Oncotarget. 2016;**7**(31):50719-50734

[43] Duns G, Hofstra RM, Sietzema JG, et al. Targeted exome sequencing in clear cell renal cell carcinoma tumors suggests aberrant chromatin regulation as a crucial step in ccRCC development. Human Mutation. 2012;**33**(7):1059-1062

[44] Hylebos M, Van Camp G, Vandeweyer G, et al. Large-scale copy number analysis reveals variations in genes not previously associated with malignant pleural mesothelioma. Oncotarget. 2017;**8**(69):113673-113686

[45] Mar BG, Chu SH, Kahn JD, et al. *SETD2* alterations impair DNA damage recognition and lead to resistance to chemotherapy in leukemia. Blood. 2017;**130**(24):2631-2641

[46] Sheng Y, Ji Z, Zhao H, et al. Downregulation of the histone methyltransferase *SETD2* promotes imatinib resistance in chronic myeloid leukaemia cells. Cell Proliferation. 2019;**52**(4):e12611

[47] Ishimoto K, Kawamata N, Uchihara Y, et al. Ubiquitination of lysine 867 of the human SETDB1 protein upregulates its histone H3 lysine 9 (H3K9) methyltransferase activity. PLoS One. 2016;**11**(10):e0165766

[48] Karanth AV, Maniswami RR, Prashanth S, et al. Emerging role of SETDB1 as a therapeutic target. Expert Opinion on Therapeutic Targets. 2017;**21**(3):319-331

[49] Kang HC, Kim HK, Lee S, et al. Whole exome and targeted deep sequencing identify genome-wide allelic loss and frequent SETDB1 mutations in malignant pleural mesotheliomas. Oncotarget. 2016;**7**(7):8321-8331

[50] Furth N, Aylon Y. The *LATS1* and *LATS2* tumor suppressors: Beyond the hippo pathway. Cell Death and Differentiation. 2017;**24**(9):1488-1501

[51] Visser S, Yang X. LATS tumor suppressor: A new governor of cellular homeostasis. Cell Cycle. 2010;**9**(19):3892-3903

[52] Murakami H, Mizuno T, Taniguchi T, et al. *LATS2* is a tumor suppressor gene of malignant mesothelioma. Cancer Research. 2011;**71**(3):873-883

[53] Quetel L, Meiller C, Assie JB, et al. Genetic alterations of malignant pleural mesothelioma: Association with tumor heterogeneity and overall survival. Molecular Oncology. 2020;**14**(6):1207-1223

[54] Tranchant R, Quetel L, Tallet A, et al. Co-occurring mutations of tumor suppressor genes, *LATS2* and *NF2*, in malignant pleural mesothelioma. Clinical Cancer Research. 2017;**23**(12):3191-3202

[55] Mizuno T, Murakami H, Fujii M, et al. YAP induces malignant mesothelioma cell proliferation by upregulating transcription of cell cycle-promoting genes. Oncogene. 2012;**31**(49):5117-5122

[56] Tanaka I, Osada H, Fujii M, et al. LIM-domain protein AJUBA suppresses malignant mesothelioma cell proliferation via hippo signaling cascade. Oncogene. 2015;**34**(1):73-83

[57] Franca R, Belfiore A, Spadari S, Maga G. Human DEAD-box ATPase DDX3 shows a relaxed nucleoside substrate specificity. Proteins. 2007;**67**(4):1128-1137

[58] Sharma D, Jankowsky E. The Ded1/DDX3 subfamily of DEAD-box RNA helicases. Critical Reviews in Biochemistry and Molecular Biology. 2014;**49**(4):343-360

[59] Bol GM, Xie M, Raman V. DDX3, a potential target for cancer treatment. Molecular Cancer. 2015;**14**:188

[60] Amador FJ, Stathopulos PB, Enomoto M, Ikura M. Ryanodine receptor calcium release channels: Lessons from structure-function studies. The FEBS Journal. 2013;**280**(21):5456-5470

[61] Schmitt K, Molfenter B, Laureano NK, et al. Somatic mutations and promotor methylation of the ryanodine receptor 2 is a common event in the pathogenesis of head and neck cancer. International Journal of Cancer. 2019;**145**(12):3299-3310

[62] Lee EJ, Tournier C. The requirement of uncoordinated 51-like kinase 1 (*ULK1*) and *ULK2* in the regulation of autophagy. Autophagy. 2011;**7**(7):689-695

[63] Shukla S, Patric IR, Patil V, et al. Methylation silencing of *ULK2*, an autophagy gene, is essential for astrocyte transformation and tumor growth. The Journal of Biological Chemistry. 2014;**289**(32):22306-22318

[64] Choi EJ, Lee JH, Kim MS, Song SY, Yoo NJ, Lee SH. Intratumoral heterogeneity of somatic mutations for *NRIP1*, *DOK1*, *ULK1*, *ULK2*, *DLGAP3*, *PARD3* and *PRKCI* in colon cancers. Pathology Oncology Research. 2018;**24**(4):827-832

[65] Follo C, Cheng Y, Richards WG, Bueno R, Broaddus VC. Inhibition of autophagy initiation potentiates chemosensitivity in mesothelioma. Molecular Carcinogenesis. 2018;**57**(3):319-332

[66] Srivastava L, Lapik YR, Wang M, Pestov DG. Mammalian DEAD box protein Ddx51 acts in 3′ end maturation of 28S rRNA by promoting the release of U8 snoRNA. Molecular and Cellular Biology. 2010;**30**(12):2947-2956

[67] Sun W, Cang S, Lv X, et al. *DDX51* gene promotes proliferation by activating Wnt/beta-catenin signaling in breast cancer. International Journal of Clinical and Experimental Pathology. 2017;**10**(11):10892-10900

[68] Taylor KH, Pena-Hernandez KE, Davis JW, et al. Large-scale CpG methylation analysis identifies novel candidate genes and reveals methylation hotspots in acute lymphoblastic leukemia. Cancer Research. 2007;**67**(6):2617-2625

[69] Wang X, Liu H, Zhao C, Li W, Xu H, Chen Y. The DEAD-box RNA helicase 51 controls non-small cell lung cancer proliferation by regulating cell cycle progression via multiple pathways. Scientific Reports. 2016;**6**:26108

[70] Zhao L, Lee VHF, Ng MK, Yan H, Bijlsma MF. Molecular subtyping of cancer: Current status and moving toward clinical applications. Briefings in Bioinformatics. 2019;**20**(2):572-584

[71] Gordon GJ, Rockwell GN, Jensen RV, et al. Identification of novel candidate oncogenes and tumor suppressors in malignant pleural mesothelioma using large-scale transcriptional profiling. The American Journal of Pathology. 2005;**166**(6):1827-1840

[72] de Reynies A, Jaurand MC, Renier A, et al. Molecular classification of malignant pleural mesothelioma: Identification of a poor prognosis subgroup linked to the epithelial-to-mesenchymal transition. Clinical Cancer Research. 2014;**20**(5):1323-1334

[73] Shen R, Olshen AB, Ladanyi M. Integrative clustering of multiple genomic data types using a joint latent variable model with application to breast and lung cancer subtype analysis. Bioinformatics. 2009;**25**(22):2906-2912

[74] Vaske CJ, Benz SC, Sanborn JZ, et al. Inference of patient-specific pathway activities from multi-dimensional cancer genomics data using PARADIGM. Bioinformatics. 2010;**26**(12):i237-i245

[75] Blum Y, Meiller C, Quetel L, et al. Dissecting heterogeneity in malignant pleural mesothelioma through histo-molecular gradients for clinical applications. Nature Communications. 2019;**10**(1):1333

[76] Lopez-Rios F, Chuai S, Flores R, et al. Global gene expression profiling of pleural mesotheliomas: Overexpression of aurora kinases and P16/*CDKN2A* deletion as prognostic factors and critical evaluation of microarray-based prognostic prediction. Cancer Research. 2006;**66**(6):2970-2979

[77] Creighton CJ, Gibbons DL, Kurie JM. The role of epithelial-mesenchymal transition programming in invasion and metastasis: A clinical perspective. Cancer Management and Research. 2013;**5**:187-195

[78] Severson DT, De Rienzo A, Bueno R. Mesothelioma in the age of "Omics": Before and after the cancer genome atlas. The Journal of Thoracic and Cardiovascular Surgery. 2020;**S0022-5223, 20**:30998

[79] Szlosarek PW, Steele JP, Nolan L, et al. Arginine deprivation with Pegylated arginine deiminase in patients with argininosuccinate synthetase 1-deficient malignant pleural mesothelioma: A randomized clinical trial. JAMA Oncology. 2017;**3**(1):58-66

[80] Kuperstein I, Grieco L, Cohen DP, Thieffry D, Zinovyev A, Barillot E. The shortest path is not the one you know: Application of biological network resources in precision oncology research. Mutagenesis. 2015;**30**(2):191-204

[81] Gordon GJ, Jensen RV, Hsiao LL, et al. Translation of microarray data into clinically relevant cancer diagnostic tests using gene expression ratios in lung cancer and mesothelioma. Cancer Research. 2002;**62**(17):4963-4967

[82] De Rienzo A, Dong L, Yeap BY, et al. Fine-needle aspiration biopsies for gene expression ratio-based diagnostic and prognostic tests in malignant pleural mesothelioma. Clinical Cancer Research. 2011;**17**(2):310-316

[83] Gordon GJ, Dong L, Yeap BY, et al. Four-gene expression ratio test

for survival in patients undergoing surgery for mesothelioma. Journal of the National Cancer Institute. 2009;**101**(9):678-686

[84] Gordon GJ, Jensen RV, Hsiao LL, et al. Using gene expression ratios to predict outcome among patients with mesothelioma. Journal of the National Cancer Institute. 2003;**95**(8):598-605

[85] De Rienzo A, Richards WG, Yeap BY, et al. Sequential binary gene ratio tests define a novel molecular diagnostic strategy for malignant pleural mesothelioma. Clinical Cancer Research. 2013;**19**(9):2493-2502

[86] Payne K, Gavan SP, Wright SJ, Thompson AJ. Cost-effectiveness analyses of genetic and genomic diagnostic tests. Nature Reviews. Genetics. 2018;**19**(4):235-246

[87] Pass HI. Commentary: Tasting individual ingredients of meso soup: Can 'omics bring out the flavor? The Journal of Thoracic and Cardiovascular Surgery. 2020;**160**(4):1084-1085

[88] Suva ML, Tirosh I. Single-cell RNA sequencing in cancer: Lessons learned and emerging challenges. Molecular Cell. 2019;**75**(1):7-12